101+
SECRETS
from
NUTRITION
SCHOOL

THAT YOU NEED TO KNOW

LYNNE DORNER
CERTIFIED HOLISTIC HEALTH COACH

101+ Secrets from Nutrition School

To contact the author or publisher, visit
Lynne Dorner | Aware of This?
315 West 55th Street, Suite LD
New York, NY 10019
www.NutritionSchoolSecrets.com

Library of Congress Control Number: 2014918663
Hardback ISBN: 978-0990915522
Paperback ISBN: 978-0990915577
Paperback Distribution ISBN: 978-1505228083
BISAC Code: Health & Fitness / Diet & Nutrition / Nutrition

First Edition Printing
April 1, 2015 version

Printed in the United States of America

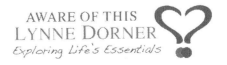

AWARE OF THIS
LYNNE DORNER
Exploring Life's Essentials

In loving memory of my grandparents,

Anthony and Margaret Dorner

I Can Only Imagine—MercyMe

Love always,

Lynne Margaret

To my baby, my legacy,

Lexington Anthony

We lived this journey together.
I'm so proud to be your Mom.
Each step of the way you celebrated with me,
sacrificed and loved me through it.
We got this!
I love you so much—
I couldn't have asked God for more.

TABLE OF CONTENTS

FOREWORD

by Marilena Minucci

What is your heart set on in this lifetime? What do you secretly desire? What would you do if you knew you could only succeed?

These are some of the juicy questions I like to ask my coaching clients right out of the gate. This way we focus on what is most important to them instead of focusing on the same old, sorry, tired goals they have had for years that no longer hold any excitement.

We all suffer from time to time with what I call "**Goal Fatigue**" especially around our health--- the "should" goals of losing weight, exercising, lowering cholesterol, etc.

Can you feel the enthusiasm? Me either.

What if instead, there was an approach that put your most exciting, life-affirming goal at the top of your list every day? Chances are you already know what this goal is but you have not dared to dream that you could actually make it happen. Do you want to live in Italy? Travel the world? Write a book? Be a musician? Have more time with your kids or just for yourself?

Big or small, staying in touch with these dream goals has everything to do with your overall health.

Creating true wellness is about a "whole-person" approach. It's about nourishment that not only comes from your food, but from every other aspect of your life and bringing all parts of yourself into harmony in a way that not only allows you to live well, but to really thrive, grow and be joyful.

The idea of becoming "healthy" can sound like drudge work, but it doesn't have to be. As we begin to make lifestyle changes, we can take a gentler, more self-compassionate and loving approach that will actually deliver longer-lasting results.

When we infuse our daily action steps with passion for something truly meaningful in our lives, we turn the "shoulds" into "non-negotiables." It's easier, for instance, to get out and walk every day or make better food choices when you can see how these activities connect you to a higher purpose even if that purpose is not totally clear yet or it is just to have more energy, less stress or to be more engaged in your life.

In any event, when we ignore our most important needs and desires, we create imbalance and deep cravings that we tend to try to satisfy with all sorts of distractions and behaviors that frankly, in the long run, do not serve us.

Are you really ready to begin? Sometimes we find ourselves putting conditions on our happiness and think that we are not allowed to ask for the bigger things we wish to have, do, or experience— **UNTIL**... "until I make more money," "until I lose the weight," "until I find my soul mate." Been there, done that, doesn't work.

The importance of all this for me hit home as I took care of my two parents until their passing only a few years apart. They both had one clear message for me: Life goes by before you know it. One day everything seems fine and the next, everything can change. Do what you really want to do while you still can. Find a way.

Message received.

That said, even the idea of wanting to make change in our lives, as needed and as exciting as it may be, can also be scary. This is normal. As much as we say we want change, we might still fear the process or the result and we owe it to ourselves to work through and get past it: If we change, what else will have to shift? How else will I have to show up in my life? What might I have to let go of or release?

In over 20 years of coaching and supporting people to make change, not to mention the many times I have reinvented my own self through life's big transitions, I have come to know a few **"secrets"** of my own about getting past these fears:

- We often accomplish more with small tweaks and taking tiny steps rather than making giant sweeping leaps.

- Change is a loving process not a "beat yourself" up fest. It's about "Progress not Perfection" and "More or Less"... **not** "All or Nothing." It's not about deprivation either.

- You can only make change in the present. Can you let go and forgive yourself for the past and try not to worry about tomorrow? It will take care of itself.

- When you spend your energy on changing you, sometimes others close to you will naturally shift as well. Sometimes they don't. Either way, you win.

- Our lives are always evolving. It is totally our choice to go with the flow or stay stuck and get dragged along.

- When you are serious about change, it's best to focus on the most important things first and get the support you need to keep you clear and unstuck. Getting a health coach is a great place to start.

- Change is not a straight-line process. There is no failure— only learning. Stay curious about what works for you and moves you in the direction you wish... and what does not.

These are the kinds of secrets I can never keep to myself because they are so worth sharing with anyone who is interested in creating a happier, healthier life.

If the title of this book spoke to you, chances are you are hoping to find something more or you simply can't resist a good secret...

- **A good secret is delicious.** You savor and hold on to it until you can't keep it to yourself anymore. You know it to be true and powerful. No wonder, the best secrets spread like wildfire.

- **A good secret reveals you to yourself.** That is the nature of the golden nuggets you will find in this book, each one offering you a stepping stone to explore what works for you. We love being in the know! But how well do we know ourselves?

- **A good secret sparks your passion.** It gets you jazzed up and can clear the way for taking action.

Secret Recipes—Secret Ingredients—Secrets of Success: All of these you will find within these pages. If you have read this far, you have already taken the first step. One more small step at a time and before you know it, you will look back over your shoulder and find that you've come a very long way toward wellness.

Let your inner wisdom speak to you. What is the risk of trying just one new thing now? What is the risk of not trying? Think what could be different in an hour, a day, a week, a month or a year from now? What secrets will you have to share then?

Let the passion that flows through these pages, inspired by Lynne Dorner's transformational journey while at the Institute for Integrative Nutrition® ignite your fire for creating your own best life.

Psst, come closer... let me whisper it in your ear... these secrets have the power to create a higher level of wellness than you ever imagined and a life you love! The time is now! Enjoy!

Marilena Minucci, MS, CHC, BCC
www.QuantumCoachingMethod.com

PREFACE

My grandfather lived until the age of 101. He lived his life in a way that honored himself and all those around him. He showed us by example how to put God, family, health, and country first. He was loyal, intelligent, and generous, and his life was filled with honor, integrity, and the love of learning and doing.

He was the most loyal, faithful, die-hard Chicago Cubs fan until the day he died, despite the fact that they haven't won a World Series since before he was born. As a child he was a non-traveling **bat boy for the Cubs**, and he even got to work as a **scoreboard changer at the ever-famous Wrigley Field** in his twenties. On my grandpa's 100th birthday, in honor of his lifelong dedication and support, the stadium displayed a sign in lights that read "Anthony Dorner Celebrates his 100th Birthday"—he was so proud!

Products of the Depression Era, he and his wife of almost 72 years embodied the saying "Use it up, wear it out, make do, or do without." They were the real deal, having had not only the longest marriage I've ever known of, but also maintaining most of the friendships from their teenage years—and they were always happy to add more friends wherever they went. On my grandmother's last day, she cleaned the apartment, did laundry, made cookies, and danced the polka. After taking care of her husband and children for over 71 years, she died in my grandfather's loving arms. Despite his tremendous loss, he lived to achieve and exceed his goal to see 100.

Socializing, volunteer work, church, and being part of many groups were at the core of my grandfather's life. When he was in his 80s he was an active volunteer at the YMCA (doing retirees' taxes) and the local YMCA nominated him for citizen of the year.

He was always young at heart, and was still driving, bowling, and playing cards at the age of 96. In fact, at 96, he bought a brand new bowling ball so he could work on improving his game. He REALLY danced the polka and the chicken dance. **I loved when it was my turn to waltz with him.** He was still investing in the stock market around the time of his death, having loved it since the age of 18. His relationships were strong and solid with family, friends, co-workers, and his "very important" card group of 70 years. I am blessed to have had such an amazing role model in my life.

When he died in July 2012, I was really searching for the right way to honor his life, to be a legacy.

I knew early on I was interested in helping others achieve health and wellness. Throughout my career as an electrologist, I have specialized in working with clients with health-related issues such as polycystic ovarian syndrome (PCOS) and hormonal dysfunction. Since opening my own practice in 2002, I have seen well over 1,000 cases of women who suffered extreme hair-growth problems and the shame and embarrassment it often brought. In an effort to support my clients, I have always sought out both technical and alternative health-related methods to assist them not only in the successful completion of hair removal but also attaining happiness in their lives.

I became even more focused on the notion of nutritional healing and other alternative therapies when my beautiful little boy entered my life unexpectedly early. Suddenly, at 33 weeks, my water broke and I lost almost all of my amniotic fluid. By the time I got to the ER, the doctor who examined me said that he didn't think my baby would make it. He was wrong. After four days of labor and two rounds of steroids, my son came dancing into the world. I felt petrified and helpless as I arrived in the NICU and they opened his incubator for me. As I held his tiny hand as he lay connected to wires and monitors, tears streamed down my face. **I promised him we were a team, no matter what.**

Ten days in the NICU were followed by several ER visits starting at 12 weeks, for fever and a meningitis scare, and a mind-blowing spinal tap. It was just the week before when I was told he had developmental delays that would require daily therapy. I vowed I would do whatever it took to help him thrive. Around his first birthday, we also visited the ER for treatment for pneumonia which I believe was the result of receiving the measles vaccination. He was struggling and almost lifeless. His first year was rocky to say the least; but, guided by a holistic practitioner and his Early Intervention team, I began my pursuit to heal him, which included herbs and supplements. The person responsible for this was a nurse, chiropractor, and nutritional coach. She changed our lives.

Four days after starting a specialized diet and detox that included removing gluten and dairy, my son said his first word. Nineteen days later he took his first steps. Such joy! His life was by no means smooth sailing after that initial consultation, but I knew for certain that his nutrition played an enormous role in his physical and intellectual development. I wanted to learn more. I remember when he gave me his first real kiss on his third birthday- there are no words to describe that moment. I picked up every book and searched the Internet for any information that could help him. My life became a quest to provide answers and support for my son—who met every one of his milestones, just not with the grace and ease as every mother dreams of.

For some time, I had been following the daily Facebook posts by my life coach, Karen Hudson, who had also been in a similar situation with her grandson, Jack. She was enrolled at the Institute for Integrative Nutrition® (IIN) and I was inspired by her journey. Already strong of mind, she was a successful business owner and life coach—but something started changing radically within her when she embraced nutrition education into her daily life. She lost 45 pounds and had gone from seven medications (for high blood pressure, high cholesterol, GERD, and diabetes) down to one. I admired her success and resolve, and wished that I too could undertake something so fulfilling and valuable. At the time, I had just turned forty, was a busy small-business owner, and a very dedicated and involved single mother. I just didn't know how I could manage the time and the cost of going back to school.

As a result of having a very clear intention, things that were going on in my life began to rearrange themselves, and pointed me in the direction of my goal. After an exhaustive process to find the very best school for his needs, my son was entering full-day kindergarten. My business moved very close to my home, and IIN was offering its program online so I could manage my own studying time. The biggest "surprise" gift was that my grandfather left me some money: the exact amount I needed to enroll.

All my excuses such as having no time or money to invest in myself were no longer valid. I was finally ready to put myself first after five years of being at the end of my own list. I began a one-year journey that opened up a lifetime of opportunities right in front of me. Now, in honor of my grandfather, I want to share the secrets I learned at IIN that not only improved my health but changed my life.

These 101 secrets are dedicated to every year lived by the man who had such a profoundly loving influence on my life. What do these secrets hold for you? The promise of a fulfilling and healthful life founded on the informed choices you make. Life is certainly full of delicious choices.

GRATITUDE

To Joshua Rosenthal and Lindsey Smith: Thank you for the opportunity to learn how to keep it short, simple, and memorable. Also for beating it into my head that it is possible to dream, achieve, and repeat. **Thank you to ALL the staff at IIN®**—especially coaches Blair, Diana, and Hailey.

To my core: Karen Lacy. Natalie Tincher. Dana Mansell, Jessica Manuel, Rachel Ruedy, Renae Stahl Jackson, Lisa Zalar, Jeanne Disturco, Shannon Batchman, Michelle Morrow and Tara Hogan. I love you all!

"Green Moms": Riley Hendricks, Nicole Fler, Caroline Russo, Shakima Jackson, Sandie Wilson Elder, Eleni Metaxa, Lucy Jones Block, and Michelle Gilmore Greenberg, as well as everyone who taught me by example along the way. You bring joy, beauty, and elegance to the healthy-mom quest.

To all my peers at IIN and my IIN family: Abbe Tesch, Kim Clavette, **Terra Milo,** Jane Savage, Shana Reyes, Markéta Edwards, Edward Love, Jaclyn Pipa, Kim Polluck, Laura McNiece, Jodi Coburn, Maritday Rodriguez, Shazia Choudri, Amy Jarosky, Susan Cathcart and the Sunday Night Crew. Also: Lauren P., Lauren C., Laura S., Linda C., Aubyn P., my Richard, sweet Libby V., Chris B., Jeri S., Karen D., Jamie J., Michelle M., Drea E., Jude M., Liz B., Shelle L., Shannon L., Kat M., and Katherine G.. **The ripple:** Jenna Fantuzzi and Kimberly Edder.

My fearless leaders: Rhonda Britten, Larissa Jaye, Karen Hudson, and Colette Cousineau.

To ALL of my Lynne's Electrolysis clients over the years: I am privileged, honored, and humbled to do the work that I love with you every day! You are my teachers. **Amber Kusmenko** - the day you walked into my office the world changed.

To My Seasonal Clean Eaters: Jackie, Kimberly (and the Concord High Crew), Yessy, Laura, and Patricia - SunButter balls rule!

In honor of my parents' fiftieth wedding anniversary: Ted and Mary Anne Dorner. To Carin, Chris, and Teddy, and their spouses and incredible children. To the entire Dorner, Merkle, Soens, and Gronke Families.

To my Calvary Church family: You are what heaven looks like!

To God: From whom all blessings flow.

ACKNOWLEDGMENTS

To my mentor: Marilena Minucci - I am forever grateful for your experience, wisdom, all your time and overwhelming kindness.

To my editors and publishing team: It takes a village. I am grateful for all the eyes, hands and hearts on this precious project. Each one brought a lesson and a blessing to the experience. It was all about the journey!

To my lawyer: Alex Gigante, thank you for teaching me about the publishing world and the importance of contracts. I am very grateful for you.

Photographer: Aimee Herring - simply amazing, you are a treasure!

Wardrobe stylist: Natalie Tincher, Buttoned Up Style - I love you!

Hair stylist: Paul Yung - you are the best! Thanks for all the house calls!

Floral designer: Mary Jane Jacobs, Bloom - an angel on earth!

Illustrator: Ayelen Lamas - not sure how you crawled into my brain every day!? Outstanding!

Logo design: Roman, SnakeJam Productions. I am forever grateful for you.

Special artist: Lexington Anthony Dorner Peterson Godspeed (Sweet Dreams) - Dixie Chicks

Cover, layout, illustrations and website design: Ali Anne Johnson, All Natural Design. You always save the day and you never left my side!

Whole Foods: Columbus Circle. Especially Earlene Giles.

The Westerly Market: Staff, especially Jeffrey Gratton.

Sur Le Table: 57th Street Staff, especially Sean and Asher, love you all!

Williams-Sonoma: Columbus Circle - love the new baby Vitamix®!

Trader Joe's: Staff, especially Stephanie.

Farmer Joe Morgiewicz and your entire family: You feed our souls!

GrowNYC: 9th Ave/57th Street team. Markella: You rock! XO

Presidential Chef: Louis Eguaras. Julius Niskey. Chef Nicholas Blackman. Kasia Banas. Ceclia Curran. **Jeff Ridley.**

In honor of everyone who is planted in Brazil in: Hope Orchard, Forgiveness Forest, Gratitude Garden, and Pioneering Pastures. Feel free to visit the website for more information on Agroforestry. www.Ciclo.org

To my readers: I bow to you! Enjoy!

INTRODUCTION

While picking up my lunch at my local soup and salad place I thought, *"wouldn't it be amazing if all of our life's choices were this easy to explore?"*

So now, imagine a salad bar, the kind where someone is standing behind the counter ready to hand-toss the perfect arrangement for you. A beautiful, clean, colorful salad bar with bountiful options spread out before your eyes. Gleaming silver bowls brim over with bright greens, crisp veggies, succulent olives, alluring fruits.

From bold and exotic to plain and simple, the flavors, textures, and aromas draw you near. You start listing your favorite toppings as they are being placed into the bowl and your eyes wander and explore the expansive choices. Energized and excited? Crunchy apples, pine nuts, and celery are a perfect match for your spirits! Or having a bad day? Sometimes those dangerously tempting croutons look big, flavorful, and perfectly crunchy.

Whatever your mood or appetite, the splendid array answers your needs and desires. Imagine that!

Let me introduce you to a new way of thinking. **Life is like a salad bar—*you can always choose what you're gonna get.*** It is time to think of your life as a salad bar, that offers a profusion of possibilities to fill your soul—food, family, friends, a significant other, hobbies, travel, exercise, spiritual practice, values, goals, and finances? How you choose from this salad bar shapes the course of your life and well-being and influences whether you feel vital and content, sad and depleted, or somewhere in between.

You can adjust your selections—like working for an appreciative new boss or embracing a walking routine—and enhance your life. And you can nourish your spirit by nurturing a joyful new friendship or embarking on a life-altering trip. Sometimes changes out of our control occur, like the loss of a job or a sudden illness—but the choices you make in the wake of such events will affect how you rebound and overcome.

When I work with my clients on their health, I share my salad bar/life analogy with them. It's the perfect prelude to two core "secrets" you should know.

1. Bio-Individuality™

"There's no one-size-fits-all diet—each person is a unique individual with highly individualized nutritional requirements," says Joshua Rosenthal, the Institute for Integrative Nutrition®'s founder, director, and primary teacher. According to Joshua, personal differences in anatomy, metabolism, body composition, and cell structure all influence your overall health and the foods that make you feel your best. "That's why no single way of eating works for everyone," he continues. "The food that is perfect for your unique body, age, and lifestyle may make another person gain weight and feel lethargic."

In *101+ Secrets from Nutrition School*, you will explore bio-individual secrets. Meaning? A secret that's ideal for some or most may not be right for you. Your goal is to discover which secrets make you feel best!

2. Primary Food™

Joshua also describes "Primary Food," the elements of our lives that "feed" us in addition to food nutrition, such as career, relationships, spirituality, physical activity, creativity, and finances. The nutritional value of your Primary Food can shift depending on your circumstances. For instance, you can eat super healthy food, but a toxic relationship robs your peace of mind and ties your stomach in knots. Or perhaps you just got the pay raise you dreamed of; now you're blooming with excitement and energy!

The concept of Primary Food reminds us that it's crucial to balance all areas of your life, a cornerstone secret for optimum health.

HOW TO USE
101+ SECRETS FROM
NUTRITION SCHOOL

101+ Secrets from Nutrition School takes you on an upbeat journey of the tools, skills, and lessons I cherished in creating my healthiest-ever life. And besides the secrets of Bio-individuality™ and Primary Food™, you also get fun facts, stats, and sweet little nutrition secrets you won't be able to resist.

Read it through or sample here and there. Either way, each secret takes just minutes to explore.

What makes it work? When you take action! Grab a secret and try it. What changes do you notice? How do you feel? Tell someone—do they get the same result? Experiment!

Enjoy.

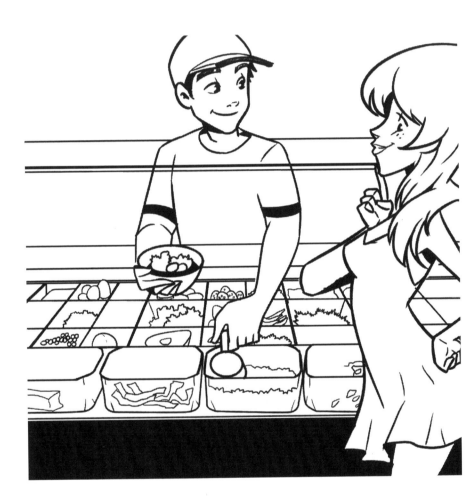

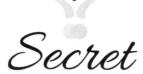

Secret

WHAT WORKS FOR ME MAY NOT WORK FOR YOU.

What's the number one secret to good nutrition?

Bio-individuality™.

This means that there's a healthy food and lifestyle combination that's right for you. Only you!

You've heard of one-size-fits-all diets? Leave them behind! What works for one person may not work for another.

Honoring your Bio-individuality means adjusting what you eat on a daily basis in order to meet YOUR nutritional needs. **You** decide what supports your physical make-up, your gender, your health concerns, your local environment, and the seasons you experience. **You deserve tailor-made guidance to make informed food and lifestyle choices.**

Do you want to consistently feel strong, rested, happy and healthy each day of your life? Unlock your Bio-individuality!

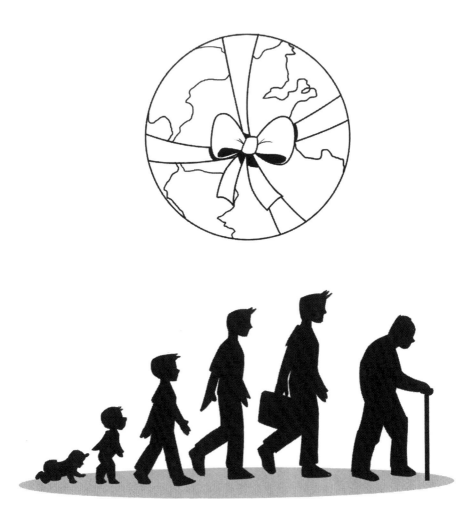

2

Secret

PRIMARY FOOD™ IS ABOUT EXPLORING YOUR LIFE'S ESSENTIAL INGREDIENTS.

There's more to good nutrition than eating healthy foods.

"Primary Food" is a profound way to refer to the major areas of your life: career, relationships, fitness, and spiritual practice. Just as with edible food, "Primary Food" affects your vitality immensely.

Don't you agree? The healthy, peaceful, enjoyable situations you create enhance your well-being, whereas stressful and harmful situations contribute to an environment that breeds disease and disorder.

What level of importance do you place on those integral areas of your life? The first step is bringing awareness to them.

To get a sense of where you are at with your "Primary Food", here are some additional questions that you could ask yourself:

- *What areas are working well for you?*
- *Do you feel like any particular area is being neglected?*
- *Which elements of your life would you like to improve the most?*
- *What would a balanced life look like to you?*

Answering these questions can encourage you to consider taking action. Write down the actions that you feel will enhance each area of your life; then do them! **As you go through this book, you can use each secret as an inspiration to take action.**

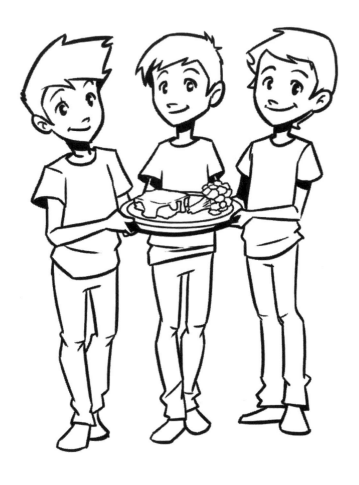

3

Secret

CHOOSE THE BEST CALORIES FOR YOU.

Many people learn from an early age that calories are units of energy used to measure food.

There is a debate that continues within the nutrition world around what appears to be a simple question: **"Are all calories equal?"**

I asked a group of kindergartners, "What's healthier: 1,000 calories of these brownies or 1,000 calories of this broccoli?"

They unanimously agreed, "Broccoli!"

If kindergartners can get it, so can you.

Determine for yourself if all calories have really been created equally.

What does your instinct tell you? In your quest to find answers, you'll come across research findings that disparage this belief. When in doubt, trust your gut and choose your calories based on what makes sense for your health.

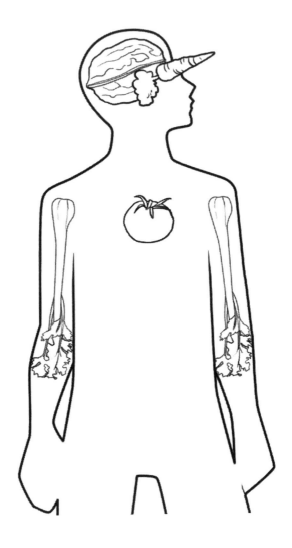

Secret

YOUR BODY IS A MAGICAL MACHINE.

Take the time to realize that your body is amazing!

Here are some facts that are just the tip of the iceberg to how amazing it is:

- Your body **temperature naturally stays at 98.6 degrees Fahrenheit**
- Your **heart never misses a beat**
- Your **lungs always breathe air in and out**
- Your **digestive system breaks down and processes** your food

These are just some of the ways your body functions, 24/7, without you even telling it to do so!

Keep the magic going! Feed your body what it needs—from your head to your toes.

You may have noticed that Mother Nature made it easy for us. **Have you ever noticed how much a walnut resembles a brain?** (I'll wait, go look!) Try slicing a carrot- it looks like an eye! Keep this in mind as you review the following list:

Brain: Walnuts
Eyes: Carrots
Heart: Tomatoes
Kidney: Beans
Lungs: Grapes

Stomach: Ginger
Pancreas: Sweet Potatoes
Bones: Celery, Bok Choy, Rhubarb
Cells: Onions, Garlic

And for the ladies:
Breasts: Grapefruits, Oranges
Uterus: Avocado, Eggplant

And for the gentlemen:
Scrotum: Figs, Peanuts, Olives
Penis: Zucchinis, Bananas, Cucumber

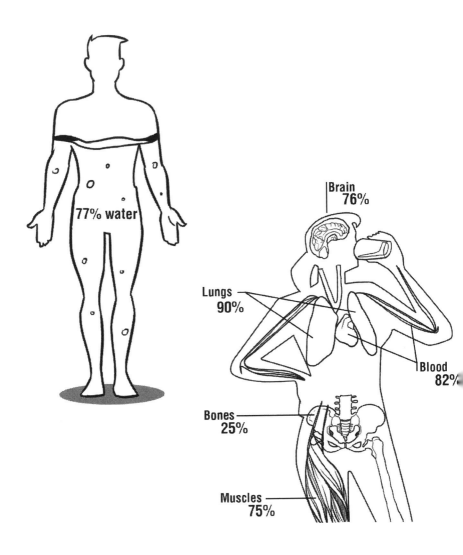

5

Secret

YOU ARE WHAT YOU DRINK, TOO!

In case you were unaware of how important water is to your body, check this out:

- Your brain is 76% water
- Your muscles are 75% water
- Your blood is 82% water
- Your lungs are 90% water
- Your bones are 25% water

Wow, those are some substantial percentages!

Since you're made up of so much water, you should replenish it often.

Be sure to consider water's effects not just on the inside, but on the outside too. Have you ever noticed how amazing it feels taking a shower, swimming in the ocean, or just running your hands under a faucet?

During those times when you are feeling a little bit anxious or stressed out, get in touch with the water around you.

Go with the flow!

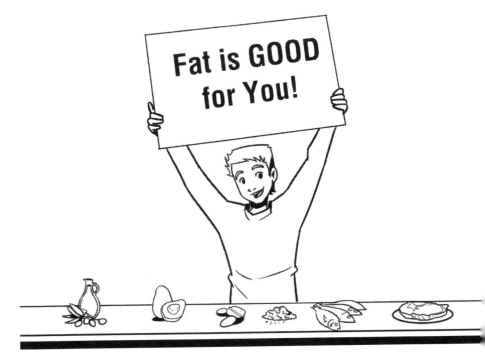

Secret

FAT IS BACK!

Eating healthy fats is good for you! Ideally, our diets should be made up of 30% fats. Since fats have more than twice the calories of either protein or carbs, the size of the portions is often smaller. It is important to be mindful of not getting too much or too little fat in your diet.

Continue to embrace the benefits of healthy fats. Fats keep you warm and energized. They are instrumental for supporting hormones, making cholesterol and keeping your brain alert.

Many people are concerned about eating fats and being overweight. Ask yourself: Is it better to consume or avoid fat? Do you buy nonfat food products in the hopes of reducing your body fat and being healthier?

In some instances, your body will be craving fat if you deprive it of getting enough. Your body can respond adversely to these mixed messages and begin to store fat. **This will cause you to *gain* weight, the opposite of your original intention.**

There is some compelling evidence that the low-fat craze launched the obesity epidemic, as more and more bodies continuously remained in this "storage" mode.

Choose these healthier fats and see if your excess weight begins to melt away: olive oil, avocados, nuts, seeds, fatty fish, or grass-fed beef.

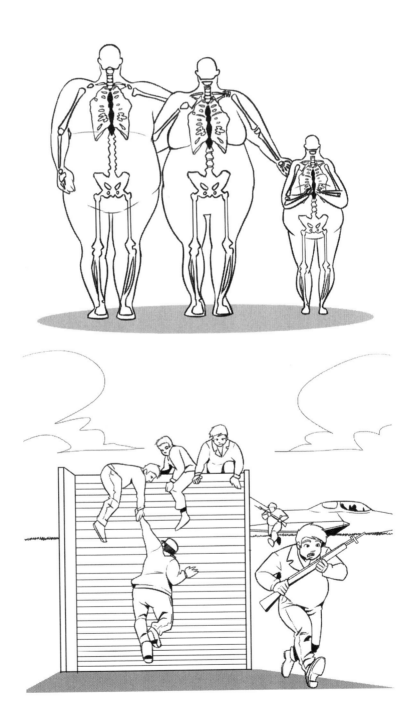

Secret

OVERWEIGHT IS <u>NOT</u> THE NEW HEALTHY.

It appears that there is a increased level of acceptance that a significant portion of the population is overweight or even obese.

Have we accepted that most of us are pudgy, and that obesity is mainstream?

I was shocked to know that the medical profession is adjusting the "normal" range on charts and in textbooks. Doctors and healthcare companies have extended what is "normal" because the majority of people in this country are getting bigger and bigger. Is this the most effective solution to have in response to this matter?

To add to this disturbing news, clothing sizes have adjusted as well. This is how companies are compensating for a clientele that is larger when compared to 10 years ago.

Instead of following along with these ever-expanding averages, strive for optimal healthy conditions as your personal parameters.

Shocking: Almost 61% of military personnel are overweight. With these rates rising, the military is worried that they will run low on healthy recruits. This is what I would truly consider a matter of National Security!

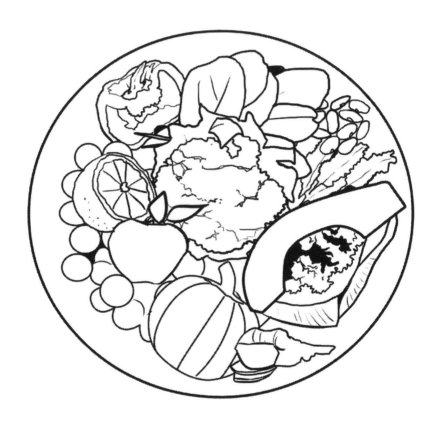

8

Secret

FILL UP YOUR PLATE AS MUCH AS YOU CAN.

Make your plate overflow with vegetables! Add healthy fruits and whole grains too.

It's a surefire way to cut junk food cravings and reduce the worry of "quitting cold turkey." If you immediately cut out foods that you've been eating regularly, it may be too much for you.

It will be easier and healthier for you to reduce certain foods gradually, especially foods that you're rather addicted to, like bread, pasta, sugar, and soda.

Focus on adding good food into your diet so you don't feel deprived.

At my nutrition school, this principle is called "crowding out." This approach allows you to feel full and satisfied with each meal. **You won't feel restricted like you do with the many deprivation diet trends that exist.**

By adding more healthy foods like fruits, veggies, and whole grains, your body will naturally crave less junk!

There I said it; you can eat as much as you can fit on your plate!

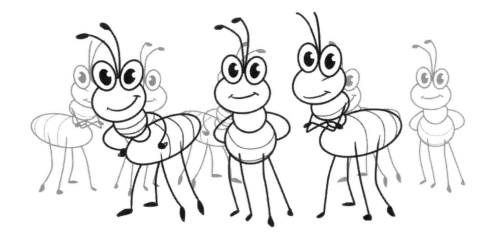

Secret 9

CHOOSY ANTS CHOOSE REAL FOOD.

I love watching ants in action. They are amazing little creatures, and they certainly have a genius way of working together.

Recently I conducted what I call "the ant test."

I dropped a piece of candy on the ground. It was made with aspartame, and nothing happened.

Then I dripped some of my organic strawberry popsicle on the ground. What do you think happened?

It was like they heard a loud bugle call and the ants came marching in tune. They were all jumping on top of each other to get a lick!

Take the ant test challenge for yourself. If the ants know enough to walk away, then do you too? If they take a bite, it's likely you could too!

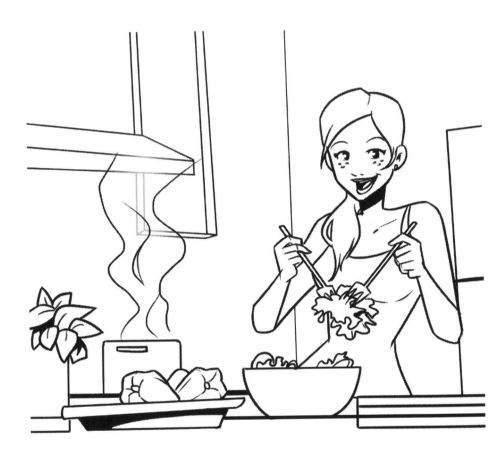

Cook for the week!

And keep it in glass containers in the fridge!

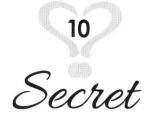

Secret

COOK ONCE, EAT A BUNCH!

Are you strapped for time? Cook once, eat a bunch! This is my **personal successful secret for producing an entire week of food options with just a small investment of time.**

Practice setting aside 1-2 hours at the beginning of your week to:

- Roast or boil a whole chicken
  (or healthy protein of your choice)
- Make quinoa and brown rice
- Roast veggies
- Cut up celery and carrots for easy snacking
  (can store in water)

Enjoy your Sunday dinner and **then use your leftovers to make soups, salads, sandwiches, or a stir fry.** It is so easy to prepare so many meals ahead of time. You know this, now do it!

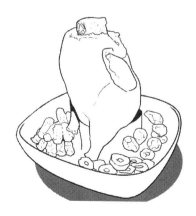

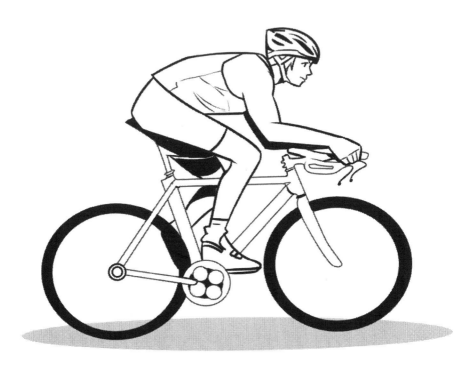

"Everything improves with exercise."

Simply ask Dr. Jordan Metzl, author of *The Exercise Cure.*

11

Secret

EXERCISE. NOW. PERIOD.

Are you still sitting on the couch questioning the many positive effects of exercise? Here are some of the benefits:

- Brain works better—less depression, less anxiety, reduced risk of Alzheimer's disease
- Digestion works better—metabolism improves, therefore helping with weight loss
- Heart rate and blood pressure are stable—you feel great and energized
- Lungs function better—healing oxygen gets pumped all through your body (you can almost feel it buzzing!)

These are our most important functions. We need all of these working effectively!

The United States of America spends $3 trillion a year on healthcare, yet is only ranked twenty-eighth in life expectancy. Something more has to be done to make up for this discrepancy, and we need to be the ones to do it.

Exercising thirty minutes a day can prevent and relieve many of the common ailments and diseases that people have. **So drop the pills and get moving!**

"What is the number-one best exercise for you? The one you will do!" Make it fun! Start with what you like, and then keep building around your routine. What are some ways you can bring enjoyable exercise into your life right now? Try some of these ideas on for size: dance while you clean the house, wash the car, play with the kids, get a Fitbit activity tracker, join a challenge, train for a race, or take swimming lessons. The options are endless.

Exercise! Exercise! Exercise! See if you can get addicted to these benefits as much as you are to your morning coffee.

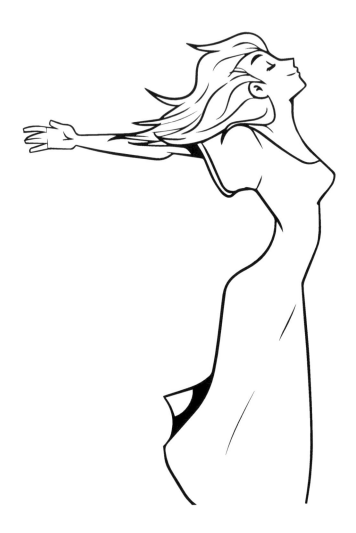

This is living.

12

Secret

THE MORE OXYGEN YOU BREATHE, THE BETTER YOU THINK, MOVE, AND FEEL.

Did you know that you can live weeks to months without food? You can live days without water, **but only minutes without air.** Yes, minutes! This startled me and really got my attention. So did these facts:

- In order to stay alive, a person needs at least 7% of oxygen in the air that we breathe.
- The oxygen concentration in our air was once 35%.
- Today the average world air supply has a 20% oxygen ratio.
- Some countries like China are hitting dangerously low levels, which will force people to stay indoors.

The good news is that you can increase your oxygen levels. Find the ways that work best for you in your environment. Here are some ideas for you to try: keep your windows open all year round, add more household plants, and go for regular walks. I highly encourage my clients to invest in dehumidifiers/humidifiers, ion generators and HEPA filters.

You may also want to start practicing breathing techniques to increase your body's oxygen intake. **Try putting your hand on your belly and see if your belly distends when you inhale**. If it doesn't, keep practicing until it does. Be aware of how much better this kind of breathing feels for you.

Try taking several quick gulps of air into your chest and holding them for five seconds. Then deliberately let out a long, forced exhale. Repeat this breathing technique three times. Can you feel the difference?

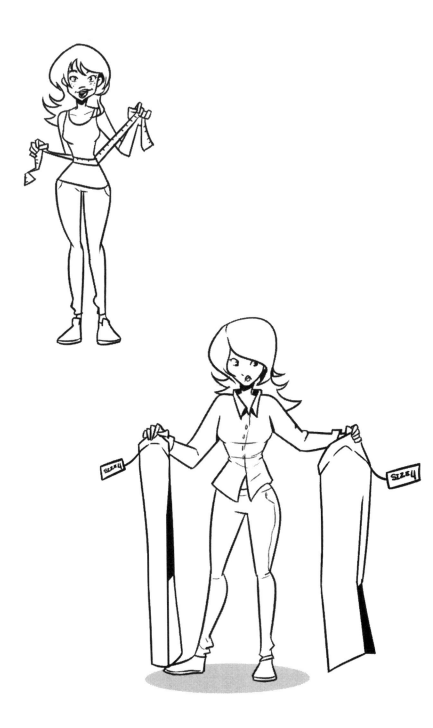

13

Secret

MEASURE UP.

Ditch the scale because it will never tell you how wonderful and amazing you are.

Do you relate your happiness and success to the number that you see on the scale? Do you have that perfect number stuck in your head? Do you beat yourself up, or rush to kick off your shoes when you are off by just a pound or two?

These are some provocative questions to consider, aren't they?

If you really want to see how you're progressing in your attempts to slim down, **then measure your waist.** Most people lose inches before pounds anyway. One of my clients was pleasantly surprised to find his belt was getting looser although he had not lost weight as measured by his scale.

Use this method: **Divide your height (in inches) by two to get your an idea of a maximum target waist size.** For example, if you are 5 feet tall, your height is 60 inches. Divide that by two. So you don't want your waist size to exceed 30 inches.

Stop trying to figure out the fluctuating retail measurements they use to determine our pants and dress sizes. Rely on the tape measure—the metric stays the same!

I must admit being a size double zero is fun sometimes but I do know that isn't really the case! And the same goes for the men who think they are a size 34 pant and their waist is more like 38.

Let's keep it real folks!

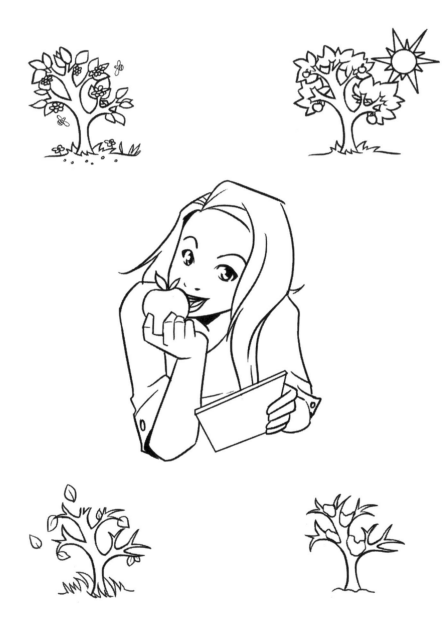

Secret 14

SEASONAL IS ESSENTIAL.

Imagine eating juicy, red tomatoes in the summer: mouthwatering and perfectly delicious!

Now imagine the dead, greenish, chemical-tasting slices of tomato they plopped onto your plate in December. Yuck!

Do you want fresh, appealing, nutritious food all year round? **Eat with the seasons.**

- Fall: Eat grounding foods like root veggies, nuts and grains.
- Winter: Eat warming, sustaining foods like soups, proteins and apples.
- Spring: Eat cleansing and revitalizing foods like leafy greens and asparagus.
- Summer: Eat cooling and refreshing foods like berries, celery and melons.

Skip the impulse to eat foods that are brought in from other places to make up for what's missing locally. Nothing tastes better than foods that are eaten in season.

Listen to your body and get in touch with the season you are experiencing. Then go get the food that matches!

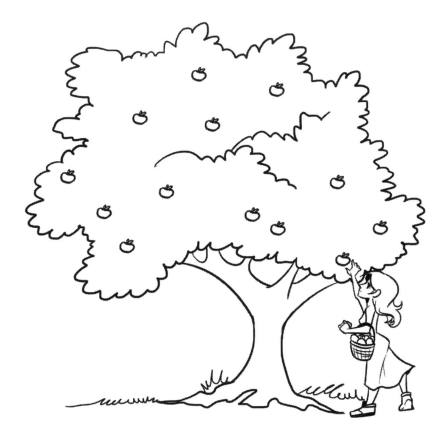

15

Secret

A LOCAL APPLE A DAY KEEPS THE DOCTOR AWAY!

Eating seasonal, organic food is great, but adding local food is an exceptional and essential healthy treat many people often overlook.

I encourage you to buy your fruits, vegetables, and meats from local farms whenever possible in order to:

- Support local agriculture by providing local wages for farmers and their employees
- Support your body by giving it the local bacteria it needs to aid in the digestion process
- Reduce your carbon footprint
- Enjoy food nourished in the nutrient-rich soil of smaller local farms which generally rotate crops

Which appeals to your senses? **A crisp, fresh, local, nutritious organic apple or an apple that has been genetically modified, ripened with methane gas, covered in pesticides, and shipped from a warehouse in some far-off land?** You decide! Now grab your reusable bags, head to your local farm, and treat yourself to the best tastes in town!

I just compared apples to apples. Now it's your choice.

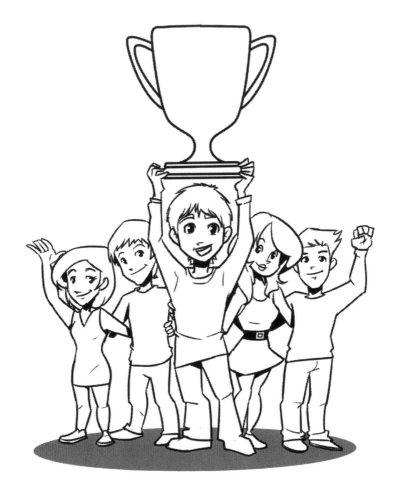

16

Secret

CHAMPIONS EAT BREAKFAST.

I admit it—I used to skip breakfast. I also paid the price for it.

If you live by the mantra "love thyself," then check in with your body every morning. Take the time to determine what your body wants to eat for your first meal. Treat yourself to a good breakfast every day.

If you take note of the key, you will unlock the reward.

What is the key? Pick foods that you love and adore. Find your mix of a healthy protein, along with whole fruits, veggies, seeds, and grains that are meant to sustain you.

Your reward? A day filled with lasting energy, mental clarity, and a vibrant mood.

Live like a champion!

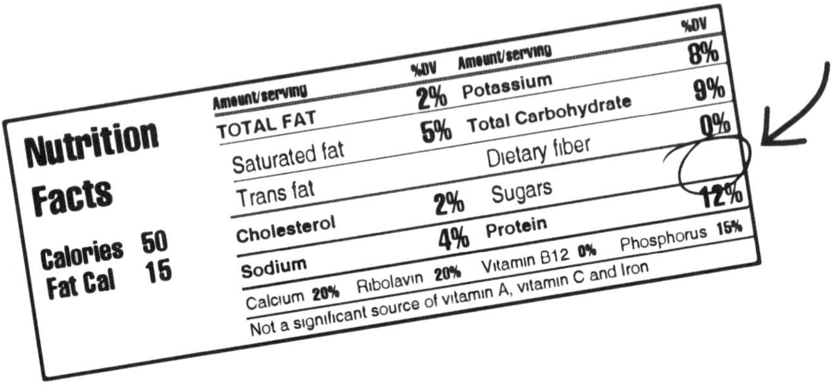

Nutrition Facts

Calories 50
Fat Cal 15

Amount/serving	%DV	Amount/serving	%DV
TOTAL FAT		Potassium	2%
Saturated fat		Total Carbohydrate	5%
Trans fat		Dietary fiber	
Cholesterol		Sugars	2%
Sodium		Protein	4%

Calcium 20%   Ribolavin 20%   Vitamin B12 0%   Phosphorus 15%
Not a significant source of vitamin A, vitamin C and Iron

%DV
8%
9%
0%
12%

Ingredients: Supercalifragilistic, hydrogenated anything, monosodium glutamate, artificial flavors, yellow, blue, red killer dyes, modified and non fat, sulfites, sucralose, acesulame potassium, autolyzed, disodium guanlate, skip, skip, skip along now.

17

Secret

FOOD LABELS ARE ONLY PART OF THE STORY.

Ever wonder what you are reading on those packages? Food labels and advertising on the packaging can be tricky. Sometimes you may even come across downright lies.

Why does the food industry hide the truth? Is it to purposely **confuse you and mislead you into buying their products?**

You may already know better, but I'd like to clarify some shopping tips for you:

- Strive to buy foods that have five ingredients or fewer.
- Notice where sugar is listed—if it is listed in those top five ingredients, reconsider.
- If you can't pronounce an ingredient, reconsider. (Let them send it back to the lab.)
- Grab whole food ingredients that have little or no processing.
- Shop for ingredients that your grandparents would recognize.
- **Don't be tricked by any claims that the product is "healthy" or "natural." Natural means nothing!**
- Use caution with foods that are fortified with vitamins and minerals.

Chances are that most packaged foods aren't very healthy, yet they make up almost 90% of our food choices. Choose wisely!

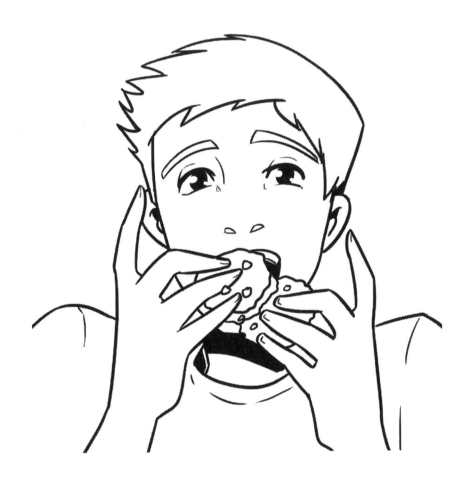

Really, baby?

18

Secret

I LOVE YOU,
BUT YOU ARE TOO SWEET...

Sometimes excessively sweet?!

Fact: In studies, rats overwhelmingly preferred sugar to cocaine. Dr. Mark Hyman explains that "while cocaine and heroin activate only one spot for pleasure in the brain, sugar lights up the brain like a pinball machine!"

Lots of people are flat-out hooked, and to be fair, it's not really their fault. The sugar industry did a sweet job keeping the daily suggested percentages OFF of the Nutrition Facts labels on packaged foods. If you grab any packaged food, you can see for yourself. The sugar information does not indicate % of Daily Value, whereas this number is listed for other nutrients like fats, cholesterol, sodium, and vitamins. But why not sugar? You know why? Because many of those processed foods exceed the amount of sugar that we should be consuming. Get this:

- Kids are currently exceeding *thirty-four* teaspoons a day. The maximum should be six teaspoons.

- On average, each American consumes 152 pounds of sugar a year. That is about 234,080 calories. Twenty-five gallons worth!

Sugar is the leading cause of diabetes, cancer, heart disease, and obesity. **You would think this would be alarming enough to demand having sugar awareness added to our food labels.** For now, you must create your own awareness.

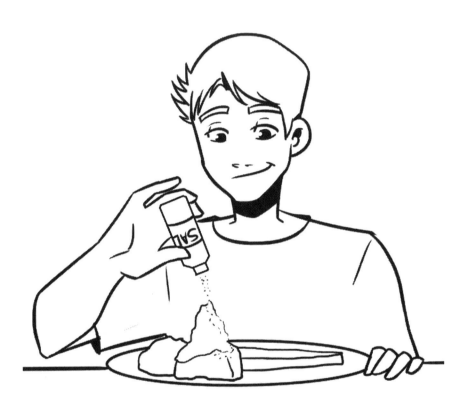

Oh, boy!

19

Secret

...AND BABY YOU ARE WAY TOO SALTY.

Salt is essential for our health, but too much can be a problem.

Excess salt can lead to high blood pressure, heart disease, kidney disease, diabetes, bloating, and asthma.

How much is too much? General guidelines for daily salt intake should not exceed 2,300 mg. Some people need less including those over the age of 50, African Americans, and people with heart disease, diabetes, or kidney disease. They should limit salt intake to 1,500 mg per day.

If you're at risk, make a practice of keeping salt off the table.

You may also enjoy exploring healthier versions of salt such as Himalayan, Celtic, and kosher. You should also consult with a healthcare professional to determine whether or not iodized salt is helpful or harmful for your thyroid health.

Extremely unhealthy amounts of salt are hiding in most packaged foods, so read your food labels and pick wisely. And when dining out, be mindful that chefs often over season their food with excessive salt because it makes the food taste better, and it masks whatever the food may be lacking in natural flavors.

Go easy on it killer, you haven't even tasted it yet!

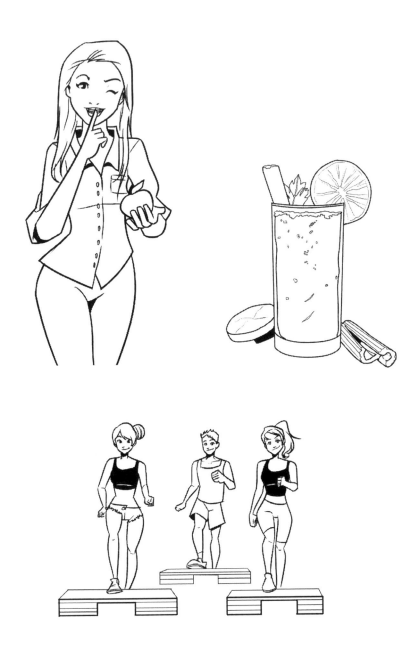

20

Secret

YOU KNOW WHAT TO DO.

You know the basic rules, right? Eat whole foods. Avoid junk food. Move your body.

Have you ever wondered: If most people know WHAT to do, then why do so many people ignore doing what is best for them?

It's because knowledge is only part of the equation. Sometimes it feels like the cabinets and refrigerator call out in the middle of the night. Or some days it feels like a scavenger hunt to locate delicious, local, seasonal foods.

Let's face it—eating healthy isn't so hard.

Creating a healthy lifestyle is primarily about making small, lasting changes. It is better to avoid shocking your system and setting unattainable goals. I want you to feel empowered!

So simply ask yourself, "What's one thing I can do for my health today?" Once you get your answer, go out there and have fun doing it!

You got this!

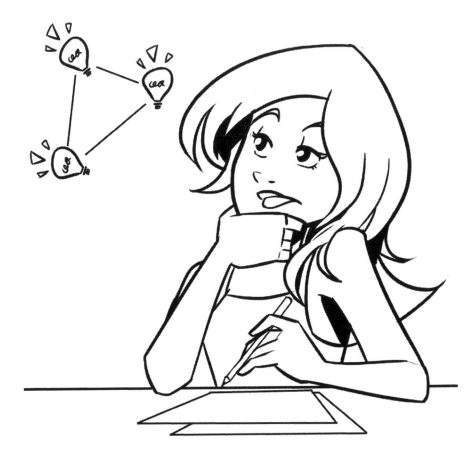

Allow the ideas to flow.

PSST... Don't forget to set your personal health goals!

21

Secret

GOAL SETTING IS THE KEY TO SHORT—AND LONG TERM SUCCESS.

Do you want to make changes in your world? Put on some uplifting music (like "Make a Change" by Michael Jackson), grab a notebook, and let's get started.

Where are you stuck in your life? What do you love about your life? If money were no object what would you change? Where would you live? Who would walk by your side?

Set goals that get you excited, goals that inspire your drive and motivation!

Choose goals that align with your vision and purpose. Stay connected to who you really are and choose goals that reflect your values in life. Spend your time on activities that accentuate how you are feeling on the inside. Let passion and purpose be your guides.

Share your goals with those you trust. Or join a group of people who are motivated to make similar changes. If you are really bold yell them out loud in your backyard or post them on social media. When you do this, you may be amazed at how quickly you accomplish your goals. Sometimes faster then writing them down.

In fact, I frequently go back to write down my goals just so I can have the satisfaction of checking them off.

Go get em! You can do this!

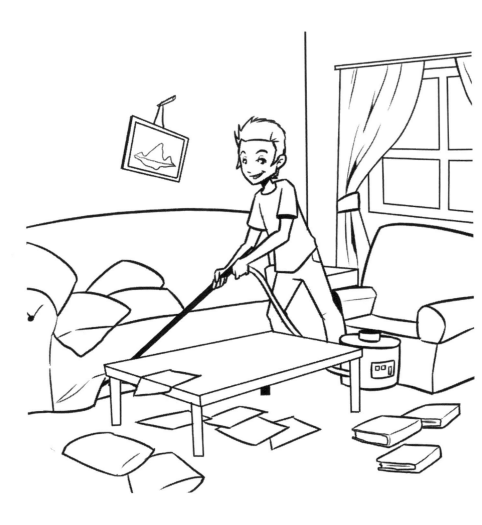

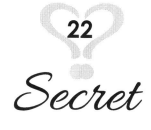

22

Secret

SMALL CHANGES LEAD TO BIG DIFFERENCES.

You don't have to take drastic measures to see big changes in your life. Taking small actions in chosen areas of your life can be extremely effective in creating lasting change.

Here are a few examples:

Home—Clean out just one drawer, shelf, or bin every day for even just five minutes and soon you will have the cleanest house ever.

Exercise—Try one new type of exercise a month. You may end up with twelve active lifestyle hobbies by the year's end and fitness will never be routine!

Food Choices—Experiment with one new healthy food each week. You'll discover that there are endless healthy, flavorful options.

Spiritual and Creative Practice—Explore one new method each month to help you find stress relief and enlightenment. You could try yoga, meditation, journaling, reflection walks, or participation in a like-minded or religious community group.

Financial Goals—Make it a new habit to save a few dollars each day. Home-brewing instead of buying your usual morning joe can save you at least $10 a week. That's $520 or more yearly toward a vacation, retirement, college fund or those to-die-for Jimmy Choos.

Simple small changes add up fast and make a world of difference!

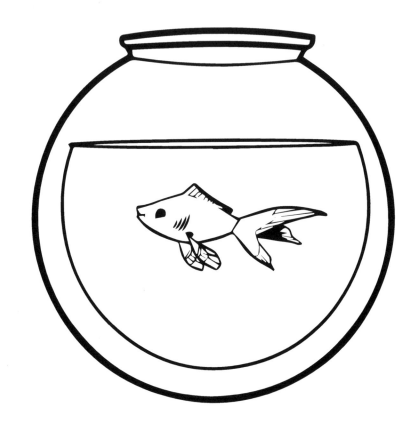

23

Secret

SAVE THE SEA,
ONE FISH AT A TIME.

We all love Nemo, right? What about your first pet fish? So cute and perky swimming around in its little bowl.

Would you ever dream of emptying your trash into his tank? Dinner scraps, disposable diapers, plastic wrappers, cat litter —poop included. That's right, put it all in there.

How is little Nemo doing? Do you think he can breathe? How long do you think he'll survive?

Now apply this thinking to our water supply. Clean water is an urgent matter for our health and environment. Water is the basis for all life, ours included.

Take a moment now to envision what is really going into our oceans and rivers—the heavy toxins, sewage waste, nuclear waste, oil, trash, and so much more.

You can save Nemo and yourself!

Be mindful of what you are adding to OUR water supply.

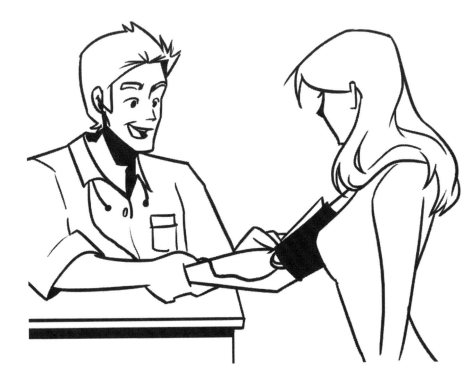

Secret

KNOW YOUR NUMBERS.

It's too common for people to rely on a cocktail of medications to maintain their health. The meds may be necessary to manage what might once have been preventable conditions. This is the real prescription: **Be proactive about your health.** Be your own best advocate.

Keep asking questions about your health! What is your blood pressure? Are you aware that 115/75 are great numbers?

Are you eating a diet filled with healthy foods you enjoy? Are you reducing your stress and creating a healthy lifestyle? How are your sleeping habits? How are your waking habits?

Become a smart patient! This doesn't mean you have to check WebMD® obsessively or find your solutions in the latest pharmaceutical ads. **Being a smart and informed patient means you know your numbers. As you strive to make healthy choices, remember to keep good communication with your doctor.**

Its time to go find your numbers: Cholesterol, Vitamin D, Thyroid, Blood Sugar — and while you are at it, find out your blood type.

I hear from my clients all that time that they are scared to go get the testing done. I was too. I promise that it is often much scarier than not knowing! Also, in most cases you can DO something about it if you are deficient or sick.

It is better to know the truth and work with the truth!

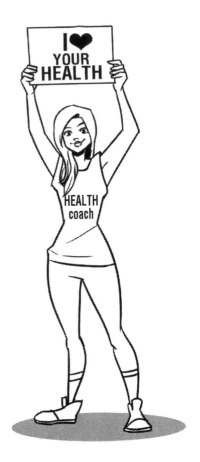

XO Coach Lynne

I highly encourage my clients to complete my clean eating programs every season for a year.

The results may be radical and long lasting—including clearing up health problems and shedding excess pounds.

25

Secret

CLEAN OUT YOUR BODY.

Cleaning out your body starts with cleaning up your plate. Eating local, fresh, seasonal, natural, and organic foods will nourish you. And won't weigh you down with excess toxins.

The best way to bring your system into balance is decrease the toxins coming in and increase the toxins going out.

Why do you need to get rid of toxins?

- There are approximately 80,000 chemicals in the world. We only know the effects of one or two percent of them. We don't know how they might alter our DNA or the next generation.

- There are, on average, 150 toxins found in newborn children.

- Short-term toxic build up can cause allergies, fatigue, bloating, and digestive symptoms and long-term toxic build up can cause diabetes, dementia, and cancer.

My seasonal clean eating programs focus on building a clean plate. This has supported my clients in reducing their toxin levels and their dependence on processed food, sugar and caffeine.

I love coaching my clients through the elimination plan which safely walks them through removing high allergen foods and reintroducing them back into their diets to uncover food sensitivities and allergies.

If you suffer from allergies, digestive issues, candida overgrowth, skin conditions, cancer, or diabetes, this plan may jump start you on the path to better health.

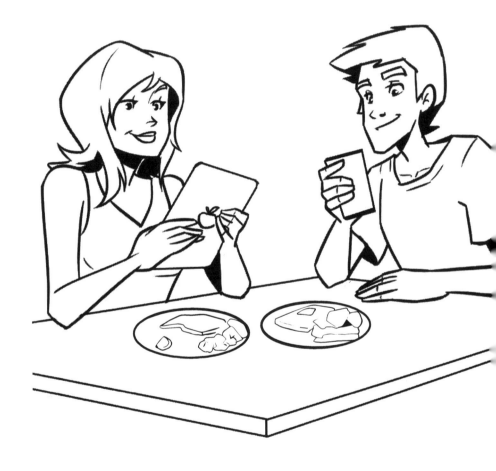

26

Secret

DON'T INVITE YOUR VIRTUAL GUESTS TO DINNER.

Skip the power cords. Practice putting the focus on the meal and those who are with you, not those who couldn't attend or your unfinished business.

Cell phones, TV, and computers distract us from our beautiful food and lead us to mindlessly overeat.

They also shift our focus away what is really important: quality time with our companions.

Create no-phone zones and savor the moment you're in!

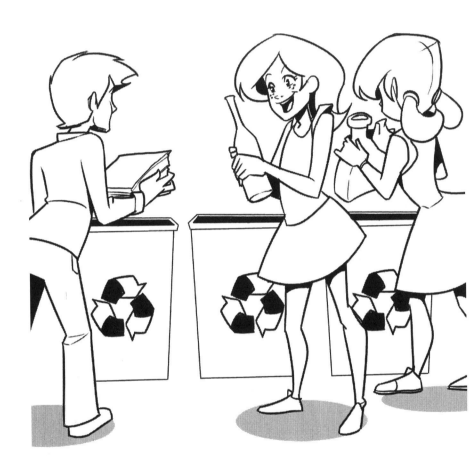

Recycling is sexy!

27

Secret

ENOUGH TRASH TALK — RECYCLE!

Years ago I realized that I really wanted the planet to be okay. I felt a strong desire to have the earth remain healthy so that generations could play outside and swim in the ocean and breathe fresh air.

Envision this exercise—Keep all of the trash you generated on your own property. Imagine the piles growing every year. OH BOY!

This really led me to think: "Why do we need so much stuff?"

I encourage you to recycle:

- ALL paper and cardboard—it is too easy!

- Textiles—yes textiles. Ripped, soiled, or stained, it is being used for insulation and other great causes

- Glass bottles, plastics, metals, and electronics

Once you get hooked on how much more recycling you have than trash, you may get a stronger sense of how urgent it is to recycle and to cut down on buying non-essential items or those with extra packaging.

The results will be obvious too! You'll enjoy a cleaner home, a clearer conscience, and **hope for a more beautiful planet for decades and centuries to come.**

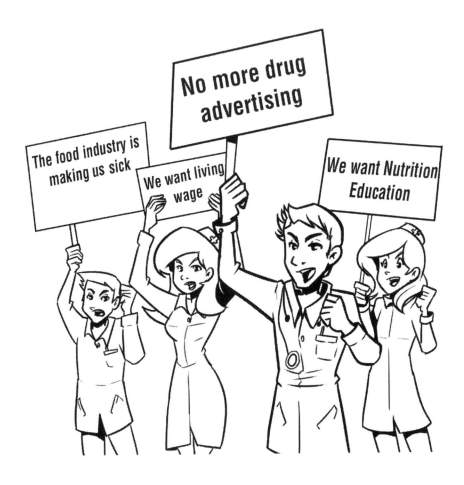

Our bright future.

28

Secret

NO FREE LUNCH.

Ever walk into your doctor's office to see drug companies have obviously supplied lots of pens, magnets, bookmarks and even toys for our pleasure? Enough already!

I am so excited that today's young medical students are starting to refuse incentives from drug companies. They want to start a revolution.

No Free Lunch (nofreelunch.org) believes that drug companies—through the use of samples, food and gifts—improperly influence the prescribing behavior of physicians and medical students.

According to No Free Lunch, if you're a medical student, here are some things you can do:

- Hold "No Free Pens" Days. Students and physicians can exchange their drug company pens for No Free Lunch pens.

- Run "Pledge Drives." Encourage students and physicians to take the No Free Lunch Pledge and become drug-company free.

- Find out if pharmaceutical companies provide financial support for medical student activities/organizations at your medical school. If so, organize a discussion to address the relationship between pharmaceutical companies and medical students.

Want to get involved in the revolution? **Leave a copy of *101+ Secrets from Nutrition School* at your doctor's office!**

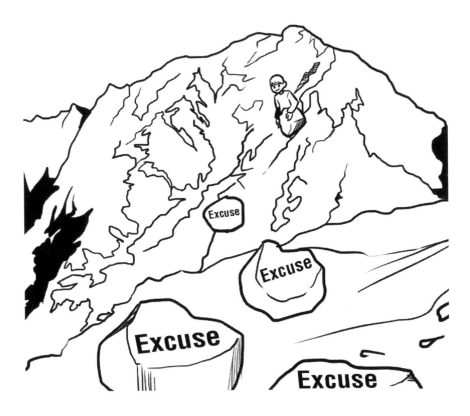

29

Secret

DROP THE EXCUSES.

Ever listen to a friend or family member explain why they couldn't get to the doctor? Or say they are too busy to exercise? Or find the time prepare a healthy meal?

This can be rather frustrating, right?

In what ways are you that person? **Think of your excuses and write them down**—ask your friends, co-workers, or family to do the same if your own excuses don't come to mind.

I made up excuses for why I didn't have time to take care of myself or have fun. I was so certain that I must spend all my time being the perfect mom and business owner. Then there was nothing left for me. Does this sound familiar? Do you have your own version of excuses?

I'm asking you to forget all that. **If you want to make a change, you must drop the excuses that get in your way.**

Once you drop the excuses, you can take small action steps that lead to big results. Then the magic comes, I promise!

Excuses are so heavy—just let them go!

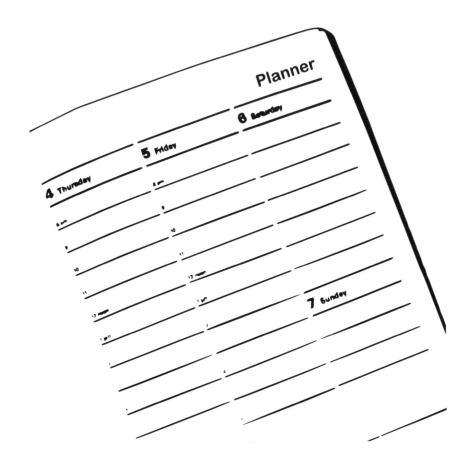

Manage your time!
Be on time! Get a planner!
Use the planner!

30

Secret

LIVE A HEALTHIER SCHEDULE.

BE ON TIME. Be effective. Be focused. Set yourself up for success. Don't put things off. This is a reflection of how you treat yourself and others! Don't waste your time—work smarter!

This doesn't mean that running late never happens. Instead, you should be wary of over-booking your life on purpose with built-in excuses.

If you are seldom late, your friends and family will be more receptive and understanding when you do show up later than expected - because it's so unlike you. Your professional life will improve as well - people will have more respect for you and take you more seriously.

Once you have mastered managing your time, you may come to realize that your bills are paid, you are getting the praise and recognition that you deserve, you are calmer, and you have become much more organized.

Evaluate where you need to focus your time to get tasks done efficiently. Work smarter not harder! Make time for things that are important!

Don't let stress ruin your day—manage it!

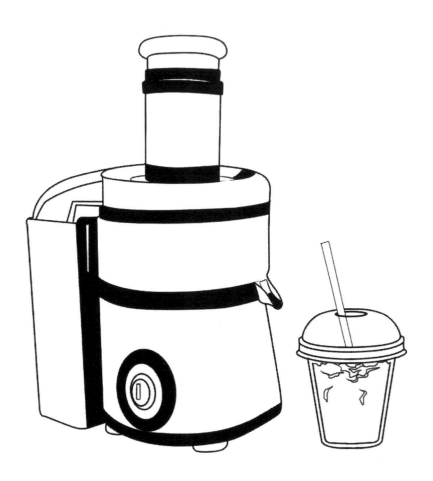

This is the juice we are talking about.

Not the carton of orange juice in the refrigerated
section or the bottles in the supermarket aisle.

31

Secret

GET A JOLT FROM JUICING.

If you feel like you're not eating enough fruits and vegetables, then juice them!

Dr. Joseph Mercola, author and founder of mercola.com, says, "It is almost like receiving an **intravenous infusion of vitamins, minerals, and enzymes** because they go straight into your system without having to be broken down."

The higher concentration of phytochemicals (you want these, trust me) in the raw juice will boost your immune system, increase your energy, and help you with hydration.

Lynne's miracle combination is apple, lemon, and ginger. It soothes stomach pain and reduces inflammation. Sometimes I add cinnamon to lower blood sugar levels, cayenne pepper for migraine prevention, or turmeric to reduce joint pain.

It's the perfect remedy if you've had a little too much to drink the night before.

No time to juice at home? I recommend that you buy fresh, local, cold-pressed juice that you drink within 48 hours.

What's your excuse? **Just grab a juice!**

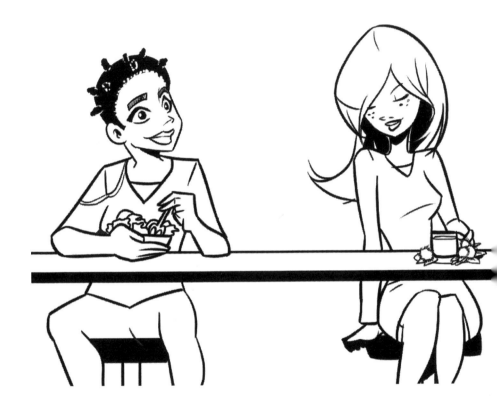

If you're a fan of *Orange is the New Black* TV Show,

don't get "crazy eyes."

Go and get your Dandelion (tea, that is) instead!

32

Secret

GREEN IS THE NEW BLACK.

Greens are superfoods! They are full of **vitamins, minerals**, and disease-fighting phytochemicals. They are rich in **fiber**, which supports **weight loss** and maintenance, and they help lower **cholesterol** and **blood pressure**. They reduce **blood-sugar** swings by slowing the absorption of carbohydrates into your bloodstream after meals. They help fight **cancer**, purify the blood, improve **circulation**, clear **congestion**, and boost your **mood**. What else can you ask for?

How about your own smog-filtering system? Leafy green vegetables are also high-alkaline foods which may be beneficial to people exposed to higher amounts of pollution in urban areas. Greens help to replenish our alkaline minerals in order to filter out pollutants. Amazing, right?

Some of my favorite greens are kale, spinach, collard greens, Swiss chard, and arugula. My goal is to have at least one of them with every meal.

This is what I like to do with them:

- Eat them raw
- Sauté, broil, or boil
- Add to smoothies and salads
- Bake them like chips

Greens can even be grown at home. I love growing green herbs like cilantro, basil, and parsley on my windowsill. I can't get enough greens. I just love them! Do you?

Did you know dandelions are not just pesky weeds? They are an amazing green plant that aids gentle detoxification in the body. Dandelions typically grow heavily in the spring and fall. Do you know why that is? Our bodies need them during those particular changes of season. Dandelions help flush sinuses and ease digestion. Roasted dandelion tea has an amazing aroma and tastes yummy, almost like roasted peanut butter.

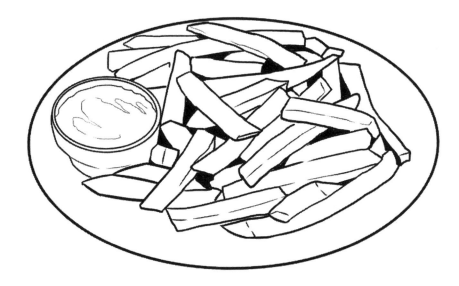

33

Secret

KETCHUP AND FRENCH FRIES ARE NOT VEGETABLES!

Yes, ketchup is made from tomatoes and french fries from potatoes, but there is more to it than that. You must consider how foods are produced and prepared. Really? Up to 17 ingredients in french fries!

Several government agencies count ketchup and french fries as a serving of fruits and vegetables. How could this be?

Foods prepared this way are food products—not food. They are often depleted of nutritional value and will adversely affect you after eating them. Remember that many of these food products are filled with **high amounts of salt, sugar, and fat.** They are also filled with unhealthy additives and preservatives.

Do you really believe these foods make the cut as part of a healthy diet?

Prepare your own fresh baked potato wedges and homemade salsa to discover how much better these real foods taste than the packaged versions.

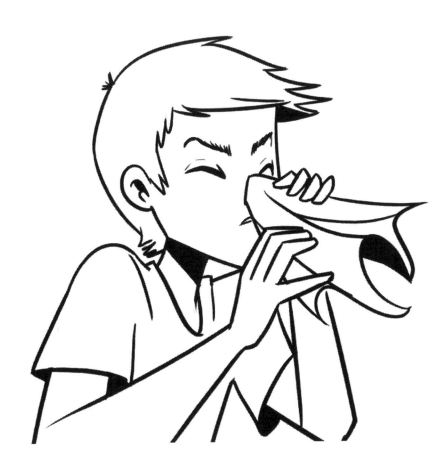

34

Secret

DON'T BE ADDICTED
TO ALLERGIES.

If you were allergic to something, conventional wisdom would suggest that you would want to avoid it. But what if you were attracted to something to which you were allergic, or even addicted?

According to Dr. Theron Randolph, a noted allergist, this is actually what happens to most people with food allergies. People are drawn to a particular food, which they eat with more frequency and increased quantity over time. Soon this behavior leads to the likelihood of becoming allergic to it.

Consider which foods you eat most frequently. Do you have the same food more than five times per week? Is there a certain food you can't get enough of? Do you experience any unpleasant symptoms after you eat a particular food?

Common food allergy symptoms include:

- Runny nose
- Watery eyes
- Congestion
- Upset stomach
- Skin irritations
- Brain fog
- Headaches

To ensure you are getting balance in your diet, you'll want to consider rotating your food choices during the week.

Here's the kicker: **These allergies may not be to the foods themselves**, but to the **chemical residues** on fruits and vegetables. We recommend to wash your vegetables thoroughly.

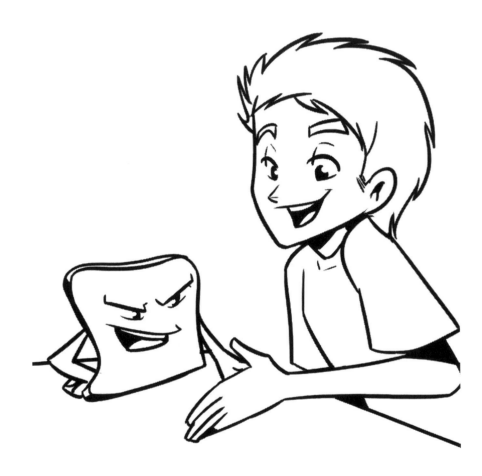

35

Secret

DON'T BE A GLUTTON FOR GLUTEN.

"Gluten-free" is more than just the latest fad. Why has it become so trendy to avoid gluten?

So what is it? Gluten is a protein found in several grains, including **wheat, spelt, rye, and barley.** Reactions to gluten can range from mild discomfort to life-threatening illness.

Celiac disease is the most extreme form of gluten sensitivity.

If you have adverse reactions to gluten —DON'T PANIC. Most likely, you don't have celiac disease, it affects only about one percent of people. Before you remove gluten entirely, it's a good idea to be tested for celiac disease (it also makes testing more accurate).

Gluten sensitivity or intolerance is much more common. Symptoms include bloating, stomach pain, fatigue, diarrhea, and pain in the bones and joints. If this is your situation, it may be worth reducing gluten to make your life easier.

You have nothing to lose. The most exciting part is that when most people remove it from their diet they feel great and many times **lose weight!**

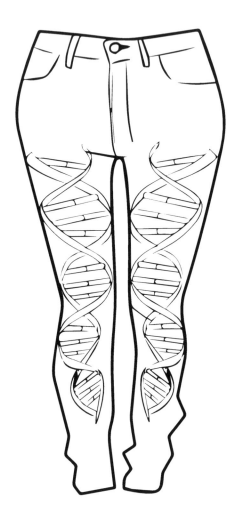

36

Secret

IT'S IN YOUR GENES, AND IT'S IN YOUR JEANS!

Figure out what's in there!

There's a wonderful component to getting healthy that includes understanding your **constitutional and your conditional** makeup.

Think of your constitution as the physical structure of your body. You are born with a specific **constitution—everything from your ears to your teeth to your bone structure. This includes the time even before birth** when your body was being nourished, formed, and constructed, and it basically stays the same throughout your life.

Your **condition is shaped from the time you are born** until the present moment. It consists of your internal life force which can change on a day-to-day basis. Some days you may be energized while other days you may feel fatigued. This depends on your daily food intake, the reserve of nutrients your body has, and outside factors like Primary Food.

The reason to consider both your constitution and condition is that your health is determined by what's on the inside, as well as what's on the outside. Through the lens of your constitution and condition, you can **determine what is in your power to control** and how to make changes for the better. Then you can **create a living environment in which you can thrive and grow.**

What are the best conditions for your constitution?

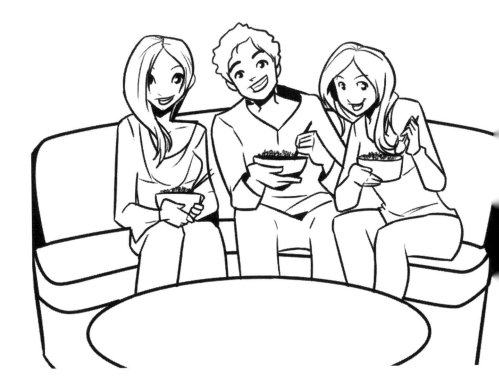

37

Secret

"GO-TO" GRAINS ARE THE WAY TO GO.

For a long time, brown rice has been the "go-to" grain. And rightfully so! **Brown rice contains over 100 antioxidants** that help soothe stomach issues, fight depression, and strengthen the immune system. It also expels toxins and is extremely versatile.

There is a perception that grains can be challenging to make. There are concerns from "I always burn the rice" to "I don't even know what quinoa is." It's time to demystify grains and see how easy they are to prepare once you give them a try. They are a consistent source of energy and they yield a lot of food (which ties in nicely with cooking once and eating a bunch!).

In addition to brown rice, there are other health coach favorites to choose as your go-to grain. Take some time to experiment with **quinoa, millet, oats, buckwheat, amaranth, and wild rice.**

Since each individual has a different constitution and associated dietary needs, you'll want to choose the go-to grains that work best for you.

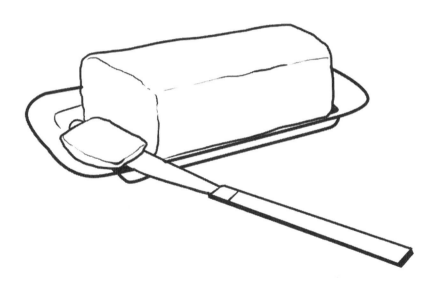

38

Secret

BUTTER IS BETTER.

Butter has been a controversial subject for years. Arguments against it are largely based on the assumption that butter makes you fat and your heart unhealthy. People easily make the erroneous claim that eating fat equals getting fat.

Where the message often gets lost is that our bodies need fat to function. Therefore, butter can assist in this process, since it is a kind of fat.

According to Sally Fallon Morell, nutrition researcher and founding president of the Weston A. Price Foundation, "**Fats as part of a meal slow down absorption, so that we can go longer without feeling hungry.**" Fat is an essential part of the mineral-absorption process, and low mineral absorption is a huge problem in today's population.

Unfortunately some people are still being told by their doctors to eat margarine, and they are heeding that advice. Instead, I would tell them to go for the full-fat organic butter.

Plus, if Julia Child were whispering down from heaven right now she'd say, "Butter is the perfect fat." She knew a good thing when she tasted it. So can you!

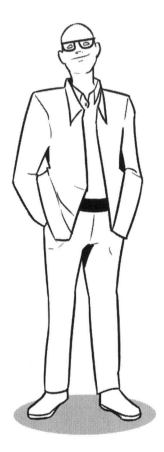

Joshua Rosenthal

Founder and Director, Integrative Nutrition®

39

Secret

WALK THIS WAY.

Have you ever watched your reflection as you are walking down the street?

I'm a firm believer that how you walk and how you carry yourself can make a big difference in your day.

Think about it, if you are hunched over and dreading your path, it will clearly show. This will determine in part how other people respond to you. It could create a synergistic effect based on how you are perceived.

Standing tall with your back straight and your head high will allow you to feel more empowered and ready to take on the world!

Be mindful to check in with yourself throughout the day to make sure that you are straight and aligned.

Research from the American Heart Association has shown that the benefits of walking:

- Reduce the risk of coronary heart disease
- Improve blood pressure and blood sugar levels
- Improve blood lipid profile
- Maintain body weight and lower the risk of obesity
- Enhance mental well being
- Reduce the risk of osteoporosis
- Reduce the risk of breast and colon cancer
- Reduce the risk of non-insulin dependent (type 2) diabetes

Imagine how much your posture and confidence will improve with your health.

Get walking and strut your stuff!

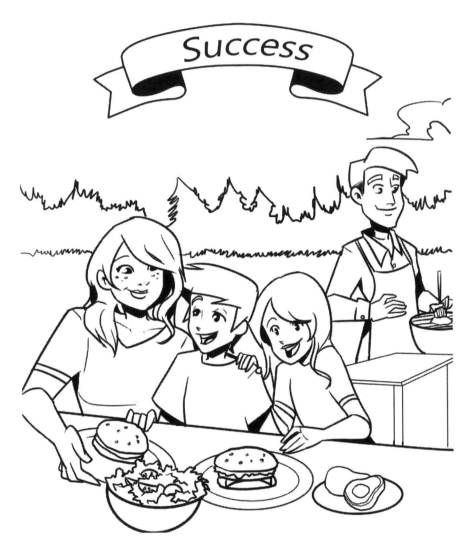

Eating according to the

80/20 puts you ahead of the pack.

Where do you stand? Where do you want to be?

40

Secret

AIM TO LIVE IN THE 80/20 ZONE.

The 80/20 rule is an amazing way of life—I first heard of this from Donna Gates and decided to tweak it as many of our teachers and instructors at IIN have similar intentions as well.

80% of the time, you will eat healthy and clean. Eat lots of fruits, veggies, and healthy protein. Then for the other 20% allow yourself to let go and add in a few of your favorite treats or foods that are not necessarily healthy and natural.

Think about the quantity and the quality of the foods you choose, both good and not so perfect. Practice these:

- Filling 80% of your plate with healthy, nutritious food.
- Eating until you are about 80% full.
- Eating healthy 80% of a meal.
- Eating healthy 80% of your meals.
- Eating healthy 80% of your week.
- Eating healthy 80% of each month.

You'll have maintained a healthy diet without being obsessed or feeling deprived.

If you eat healthy, organic, local, seasonal, nutrient-dense foods 80% if the time, you will be one of the healthiest people out there! **Most people eat processed food out of a box or a bag 90% of the time**. Now, more than ever before, these food products include GMOs and factory-farmed animals.

Joshua Rosenthal, founder of IIN®, takes this way of thinking one step further with his 90/10 rule. Now that's something to strive for!

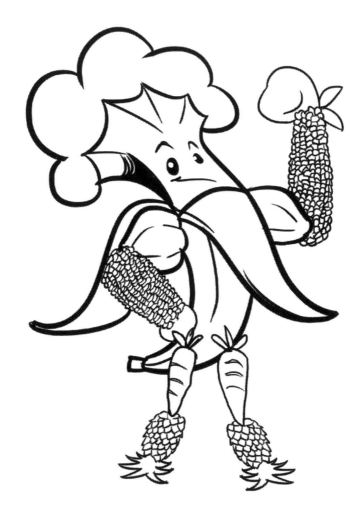

41

Secret

SUPERFOODS FOR SUPERPOWERS!

Did you ever wonder why superfoods are so super anyway?

Superfoods have disease-fighting nutrients that help keep your body and its immune system in check. Have you ever wondered how Superwoman got her powers? I like to imagine she was making her way through her own superfoods list.

Here are my favorite superfoods, including foods that you've likely heard of and hopefully have access to:

1. Blueberries	6. Cauliflower	11. Kale
2. Avocados	7. Red bell peppers	12. Lemon
3. Spinach	8. Beans	13. Apple
4. Broccoli	9. Oats	14. Ginger
5. Chocolate (!)	10. Pumpkin	15. Sardines

Okay, don't gag with that last one. Sardines are really good if you hold your nose, lean to the left and stand on one foot! Whatever it takes to feel super!

Here are some exotic superfoods that I learned about at nutrition school. I dare you to try a new one each month and see how you feel:

1. Raw cacao	6. Camu powder	11. Chia seeds
2. Goji berries	7. Bee pollen	12. Quinoa
3. Maca powder	8. Sea vegetables	13. Açai
4. Hemp products	9. Medicinal mushrooms	14. Moringa
5. Spirulina	10. Aloe vera	15. Manuka honey

Pick one of these and try it today!

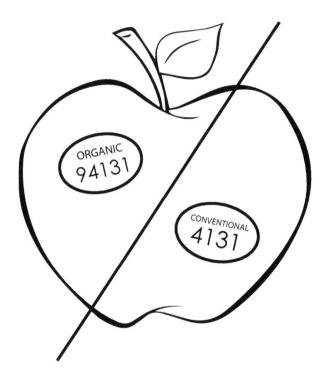

42

Secret

YOU DON'T HAVE TO BUY EVERYTHING ORGANIC.

Do you need a good gauge to help you plan your shopping? Here's what I like to use!

The Environmental Working Group created a list called the Dirty Dozen™. This list consists of the foods that are the most riddled with pesticides.

The Dirty Dozen™:

1. Peaches
2. Apples
3. Sweet bell peppers
4. Celery
5. Nectarines
6. Strawberries
7. Cherries
8. Pears
9. Grapes
10. Spinach
11. Lettuce
12. Potatoes

The Environmental Working Group also provides a list called the Clean Fifteen™, the least contaminated with pesticides.

The Clean Fifteen™:

1. Avocados
2. Sweet corn
3. Pineapple
4. Cabbage
5. Sweet peas (frozen)
6. Onions
7. Asparagus
8. Mangoes
9. Papayas
10. Kiwis
11. Eggplant
12. Grapefruit
13. Cantaloupe
14. Cauliflower
15. Sweet potatoes

What can this mean for you? You can be a more efficient shopper! If you find that you have some limitations regarding which foods you can buy organic, just make sure your organic choices are from the Dirty Dozen™. If you have to rely on buying some conventionally grown food, then go with the safest bets that are listed on the Clean Fifteen™. Visit ewg.org yearly for their updated list.

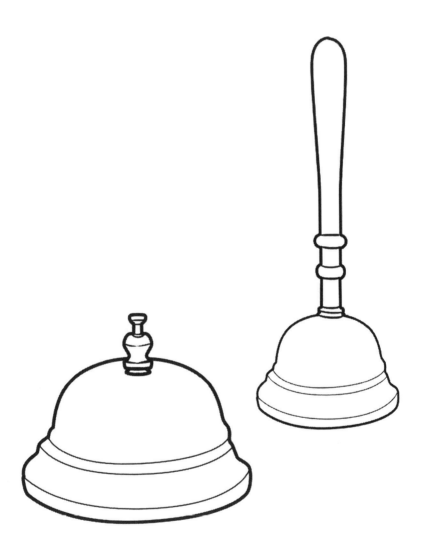

43

Secret

TIMING MATTERS.

Do you wake up naturally? Do you rise with the sun?

The practice of Ayurveda, a 5,000-year-old system of natural healing, places a strong emphasis on timing, especially relative to meals.

Breakfast literally means "**break the fast.**" The name itself reminds us that the fast is broken after giving the digestive tract a fairly long break. Also, take into consideration that this meal should be big enough to tide you over until your midday meal, but with easy-to-digest nutrients. Remember, you want to ease your digestive system gently into your day.

Lunch should be the large, midday meal that is best served between 10 a.m. and 2 p.m. I encourage clients to think of it as the "farmer meal." You are eating to sustain your workload for the day. Use what is local and seasonal from the land around you. It's also when you should have your dessert! (Chocolate with your lunch, anyone?)

Dinner, sometimes called **supper,** should be thought of as the **supplemental meal.** Keep in mind that you don't want anything too heavy. You want to be kept full until breakfast, but you don't want your body to work too hard at digestion. Therefore, do your best to finish eating by 8 p.m.

Enjoy water or tea before bed. Strive to go to sleep when the natural light has gone down!

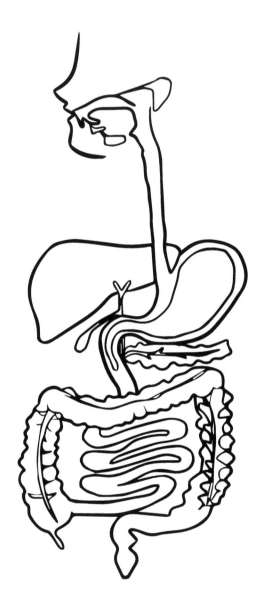

44

Secret

GET ON THE INTESTINAL TRACT.

There are so many interesting facts about the body! Did you know that the gastrointestinal tract is 30 feet long from the mouth to the anus? It usually takes between 24 and 72 hours for food to travel through your digestive system.

The small intestine's job is to break down food. It's located near your belly button and it's about the size of your fist, yet unraveled, it would measure about 20 feet long!

The large intestines form your stool. If the large intestine were stretched out, it would be about 10 feet long. In the body, it surrounds the small intestine.

Here are some essentials to help keep your tract on track:

- **Fats**—keep you full.

- **Carbohydrates**—digest the fastest and give you energy.

- **Fiber**—slows digestion down so you feel fuller longer.

- **Bacteria**—are responsible for keeping it all in balance.

Be mindful of the emotional component too! Sadness and fear can slow down movement; aggression and anger can speed up movement.

Enjoy the ride.

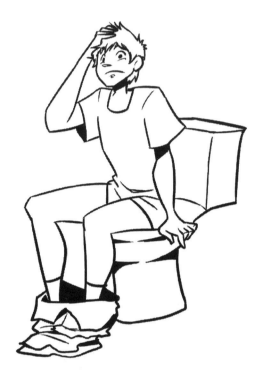

Did you know that your poop says a lot about you? If you poop within the first hour of the day, this is an indicator of good digestion and stable overall health.

Here are some funny little digestion facts that will stir up interesting conversation for elementary school kids or your next dinner party:

- The average person farts 14 times a day.

- Farts can reach the speed of 10 feet per second.

- Farting does not discriminate: Men and women produce an equal amount of gas.

Secret 45

STOP PUSHING
FOR POOPY PEBBLES.

Here's the scoop on your poop!

Do you have the constipation blues? Anyone with this problem can tell you that it feels like hell has to freeze over in order to get out a little pellet of poop joy.

Joking aside, constipation can be a serious issue. It can be due to a bacterial imbalance, lack of nutrients in your diet, like iron, calcium, magnesium, and fiber. It can also be due to lifestyle components like lack of exercise or low hydration.

One way to ensure you are "regular" is to incorporate organic probiotics and enzymes into your diet. Taking natural enzymes will help keep you running smoothly, efficiently, and regularly. Can you see how this could be life changing?

The **probiotics** found in yogurt are not always alive and can be from unreliable sources, of varying strains, and differing strength. Plus, yogurt doesn't agree with every person's Bio-individuality. Therefore, choosing a probiotic supplement can be a better option.

Enzymes aid in the breakdown of food during digestion. The good news is that whole foods generally contain natural enzymes that can do this. The bad news is too many processed food choices will hinder this process. If you don't want to take a supplement to help break down your food, **stick with eating whole foods.** Try some papaya and pineapple they contain natural enzymes.

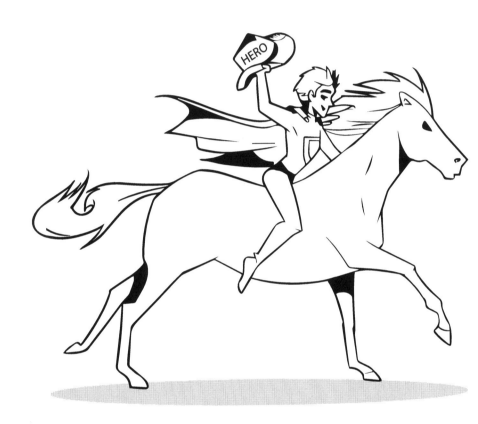

Go Howard, Our Hero!

46

Secret

BE A HERO.

Howard Lyman had a one in a million chance of beating spinal cancer. He did.

His story has much to offer us. He's a former factory farmer and meat eater who turned vegan. In thinking his dad was "old school" for being a more organic farmer, Howard made the decision to turn his farm into a $30 million industry. Big business brought him big equipment and big chemicals, and soon big sickness. After his cancer diagnosis, he realized his illness was due to the chemicals he was exposed to on his farm. He vowed to return to non-chemical means of farming if he beat the disease.

He was catapulted to notoriety for appearing on **Oprah and sharing big-farming secrets, including the shocking news that animals** had been fed other sick animals. This revelation stirred a deeper awareness of how unhealthy farming practices in the U.S. could lead to the spread of mad cow disease globally.

What was even more shocking was that Howard and Oprah were nearly silenced for bringing this discussion to TV. They spent years in and out of court for being honest about the facts, but for them it was worth it.

He and his doctors believed his rare cancer stemmed from the chemicals he used on the farm, and he continues to speak out passionately in his books and in politics about healthy farming practices.

Howard became known as the Mad Cowboy. He faced the truth and he beat the odds!

Be a hero, stand up for what you believe in.

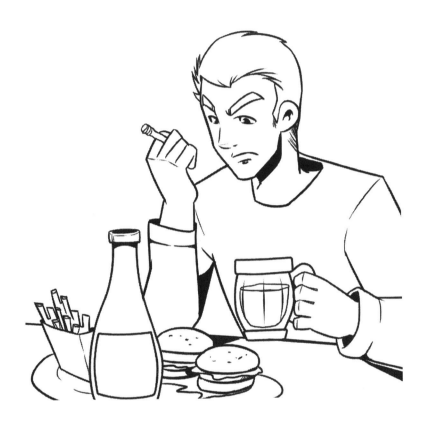

"Addictions aren't someone's problem. Addictions are the solution to a problem and the unresolved pain."

— Dr. Christiane Northrup

Secret 47

EMPTY THE ANGER
FROM YOUR LIVER.

In Eastern medicine the liver is often referred to as the "seat of anger." And who would blame it for being angry? It's the primary detoxifier for everything we eat, drink, inhale, or absorb. It has to combat processed food, pollutants, and toxins.

If your liver is angry, feed it well with foods that support it, like kale, garlic, red beets, avocados, lemons, apples, olive oil, and walnuts. Avoid unhealthy foods like alcohol, fried foods, and salty foods. Drink lots of water to flush out toxins.

Aside from feeding your liver well, you can improve its health through stress relief and anger management techniques.

It is believed in Chinese medicine that anger (especially suppressed anger) injures the liver. The liver is the most emotion-sensitive organ and its weakness is often connected to emotional sensitivity. If you habitually bury your anger, it is bound to affect the health of your liver.

What can you do with all the anger stored in your liver? Get it OUT of your SYSTEM.

Exercise. Sweat it out through kick-boxing or running. It is also essential to sweat it out during relaxation techniques like taking a sauna, being under infrared lights or lying out in the sun.

Talk about your feelings and why you are angry.

Take deep breaths and imagine releasing the anger with each exhale.

Practice this exercise: **Make crazy growling noises**. You'll notice shortly after that you feel happier. If you do it again, you may even start laughing. **This is the joy of pent up anger being released.**

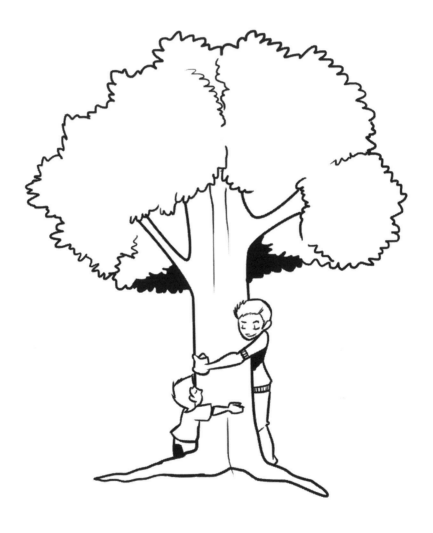

48

Secret

HUG A TREE UNTIL YOU EMBRACE NATURE.

If you're looking to embrace nature, then do it literally—hug a tree! Roll around in the soft green grass.

Did you know that scientific proof is being gathered about this? Studies show that there are significant physiological and psychological health effects on those who interact with plants and trees.

Intuitively, you know that nature is an essential element of good health and well-being. When you are present with plants, trees, earth, and water, it shifts your energy toward the positive. It's the perfect antidote to get you out of any funk.

How can you connect with Mother Nature in a simple way? Take a walk in a park, put your hands in the dirt, walk around barefoot in the grass, or roll down a hill like you did as a child.

Seriously, I hugged a tree and it felt amazingly good!

Try it for yourself!

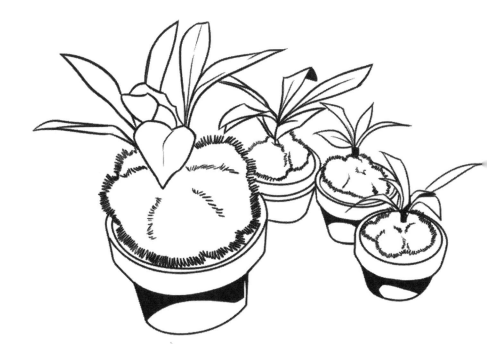

49

Secret

DANCE WITH YOUR PLANTS!

Most household plants help provide better quality air to help you breathe. Did you know that there's a symbiotic relationship that occurs between you and your plants? Why not reap those rewards!

Plants are a positive influence on many levels.

Environmentally, they detoxify the air by absorbing pollutants and odors. Aesthetically, they look attractive and add a sense of natural style (especially when you say hello and remember to water them). Metaphysically, they are meditative and help reduce stress when you tune in to their beauty.

Take inventory of your living space and determine how plants can fit into your home.

For best results, you can lovingly arrange two plants for every 100 square feet of interior space (with approximately eight-to ten-foot ceilings).

Arrange your grouping of these oxygen-boosting powerhouses: spider plant, peace lily, bamboo palm, snake plant, rubber plant, aloe (also handy for first-aid), English ivy, philodendron, red-edged dracaena, and golden pothos.

This is an easy way to bring life to your home or office. You can even share the joy—bring one to your best friend too!

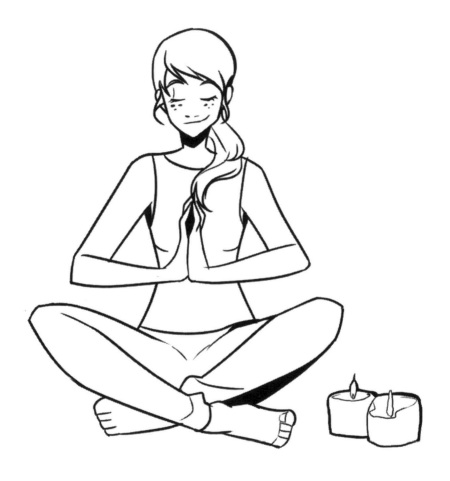

50

Secret

VISUALIZE YOUR FUTURE — MANIFEST YOUR DREAMS!

I've studied a number of visualization techniques, and use them to envision my future. Here's one to help you manifest your dreams. You can record yourself reading it or close your eyes and have a friend or partner read it to you!

*Put one hand on your **heart**—this is the center of your love.*

*Put one hand on your **belly**—this is center of your confidence.*

Take care of you. Love you. Love every second of your journey.
Live in the now.

Take deep breaths in and out.
Think of everything you are grateful for.
Appreciate who you are.

Feel the warmth and love you are sending to the top of your head. Through your body, down your legs to your feet, down your arms to your hands. Across your face to the tip of your nose.

Imagine every part of your body becoming filled with gratitude, love, and confidence.

Now is the time.

Think these thoughts:

I am grateful for all that I am.
I have so much to look forward to.
I desire happiness and success.
This is the right time and the right place.
I am loved.
My life is truly a blessing.

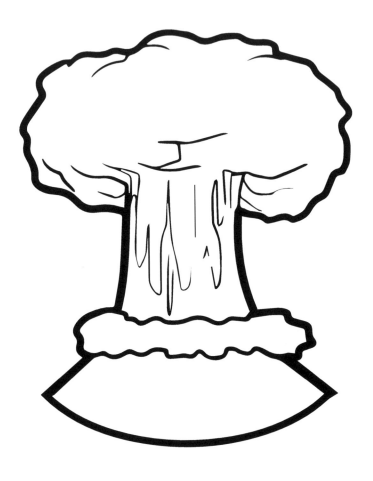

51

Secret

BEWARE THE
"SECRETS OF MASS DESTRUCTION"

While this book is meant to be positive and uplifting, these dirty secrets will shock you with the truth about our food system. I believe that it is our right as human beings to know where our food comes from and how it's being altered.

Here are some of the dirtiest secrets that the food industry does NOT want you to know:

DROP THE TRANS-FATTY ACID

Trans fat is artificially created to give food products a longer shelf life. Research studies have proven trans fat to be hazardous, but the food industry uses it anyway.

Top government experts agree that there is no safe level of trans fat, yet the FDA allows companies to put up to .5 milligrams per serving in a product and still claim that a product has zero trans fat. All those half milligrams add up and you would never know how much you are eating! Not okay! Eating trans fats increases your risk for stroke, heart disease, and type-2 diabetes. The food industry is counting on our ignorance so they can keep raking in huge profits at the expense of our lives.

It's time for some serious action in the U.S. We vote with our dollars and we **vote with our forks**. Stay far away from foods that include partially hydrogenated oil, the major source of trans fat.

GMOS, OR GM-NO'S

GMO is abbreviated for genetically modified organism. The food industry justifies altering our food supply in order to create "foods" that are more resilient. This is a decision based on profit, not on health. An example of a GMO food is a tomato breed that has had insecticidal toxins injected into the plant to produce a crop that won't rot or attract bugs.

We must fight for GMO labeling—$100s of millions are spent against the labeling of GMOs. It is estimated that 90% of people wouldn't buy foods that are labeled as Genetically Modified. Why is it okay for them to have more rights to make money then our rights to know what we are eating?

Food allergies have increased since the invention of GMO foods. Many indications have been made that animals die when they graze on GMO cotton—at the very least, where are the bees going? They are dying off because of GMOs and pesticides that are being sprayed on their food sources.

If animals and bees are dying, imagine what's slowly happening to us?

The largest GM crops in America are corn, soy, cottonseed, canola, and sugar beets. Remember, you can just say NO!

SODA'S THE NEW CRACK

The soda industry has its strategy down to a science. Ever wonder why soda doesn't quench your thirst? Because it can't! And the soda industry is very aware of this!

Drinking a 20-ounce regular soda is like eating approximately 20 packets of sugar. Sugar is the only ingredient that has no RDA listed on food labels—because if you saw that you were drinking well over 400% of your daily allowance, you might reconsider. And guess what? The food industry doesn't want you second-guessing their addictive sweets.

Studies have shown that rats prefer sugar to cocaine. Is there any question that this is a problem? Find the alternative that works for you.

P.S. Do you think diet sodas are a better alternative? They contain artificial sweeteners that trick your brain into wanting more food.

FRANKENFISH

Did you know that farmed salmon is injected with orange dye because otherwise they'd be gray? Other fish are being genetically modified to grow to twice the normal size. What is going on here?

Many farm-raised fish are inbred and kept in small, unhealthy spaces. They are usually fed chemicals to combat fungal, parasitic, and bacterial infections. They often eat other fish and each other's waste. These are not conditions for health – for the fish or for us!

I encourage you to choose wild-caught fish. Tell your restaurants and grocers that you don't want Frankenfish!

FACTORY-FARMED MEAT

A harsh truth is that most meat in the United States is factory farmed. This means that animals are inhumanely treated and raised in sub-par living conditions, fed GMO grains and possibly each other!

Factory farmed animals are most likely pumped with hormones and antibiotics to survive their brutal living conditions. Have you considered how many of these hormones and chemicals get transferred to the consumer?

If you are concerned about eating clean, you must choose meat from cattle raised humanely. The food industry has already made their choice to place their profits above our health.

Are you pissed off yet? I am! What can we do? Let our choices tell the government and the food industry what we want.

Vote with your fork!

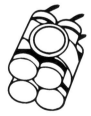 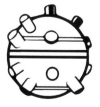 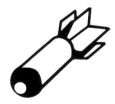

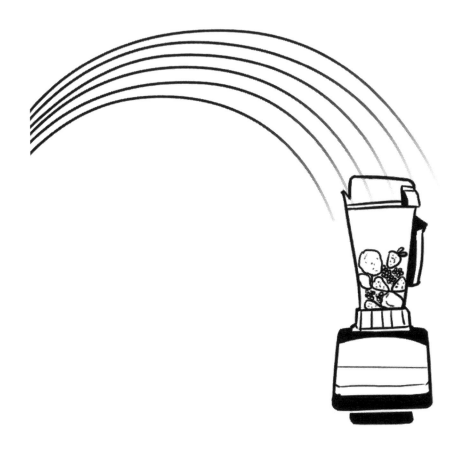

Imagine what can go in here.

52

Secret

GREEN SMOOTHIES CAN ROCK YOUR WORLD.

A few months into nutrition school, I was given an assignment to try a green smoothie full of kale and hemp seeds. I was nervous. I put the ingredients into the blender and turned it on. I thought it was too "green" to drink, yet, I did it!

With one sip, I was hooked. I couldn't even taste the perfectly blended greens, and I felt a quick increase in energy.

It wasn't until I tried it that I learned that green smoothies are an excellent way to start the day!

Here's a quick and easy recipe:

Lynne's Green Goddess

- 1 banana
- 2 Tbsp. hemp seeds (they're delicious)
- 1 cup kale
- ¾ cup almond milk
- 1 tsp. pure vanilla extract

Blend ingredients and enjoy!

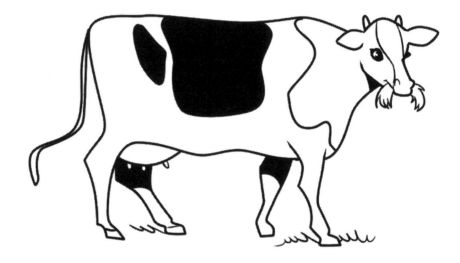

53

Secret

CHEW LIKE A COW!

I used to have a negative reaction to anyone who chewed like a cow. After going to nutrition school, I now realize those people are likely healthier for it!

Do you like to chew? Have you ever pondered this? Chewing is so automatic that you may take it for granted.

The benefits are incredible. **Digestion starts in the mouth** with the release of saliva to start breaking down your food. Whether solid or liquid, food is meant to be chewed and chewed thoroughly.

I encourage you to chew and swish around your smoothies. Slow down and be mindful of your chewing, and you will enjoy your food more. Rediscover the gratification of this basic practice and feel the profound effects on your health.

Go ahead, chew like a cow!

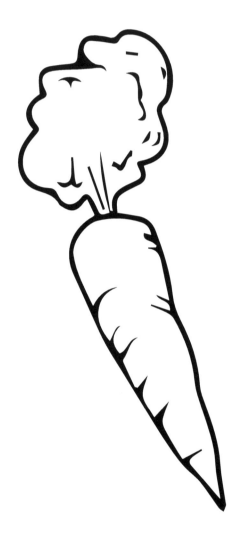

54

Secret

TO COOK OR NOT TO COOK? THAT IS THE QUESTION.

I recently chomped on some raw corn on the cob. It was delicious! I highly recommend this wonderfully fresh, crisp treat (just make sure it's non-GMO).

In the winter time, there is nothing like a warm stew or a hot soup. In the summer, it's all about the cooling effects of raw fruits and veggies.

Most people enjoy a mix of raw and cooked foods. However, many raw food advocates believe that food is best eaten in its natural unprepared state, with all the enzymes intact. But practitioners of traditional Chinese medicine believe that cold, raw foods require too much energy from the body to digest, and put a damper on the body's digestive fires. They believe that over time, this can weaken the body's digestive system, causing bloating, flatulence, and poor absorption of the nutrients in foods.

If you want to pack your diet with the natural enzymes and nutrients found in raw food, then go with it. If you feel you need cooked foods for proper absorption or protection, then honor your decision. But **you don't need to make such a black-and-white choice about how to eat your food.** You can choose your own combination based on how certain foods make your body feel. This is how to listen to your bio-individuality.

What are **your** needs?

What is the best ratio of raw and cooked foods for you?

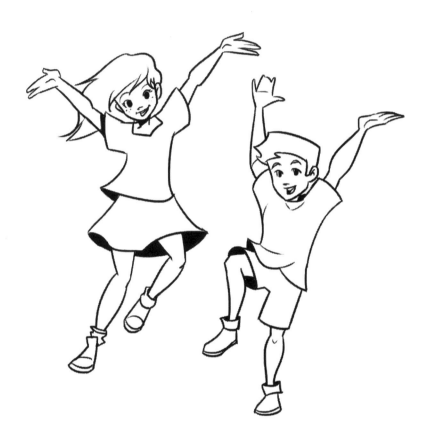

55

Secret

YOU CAN DO THE HOKEY POKEY AND TURN YOURSELF AROUND.

Sing along with me! You put your veggies in, you take the sugar out...You put your veggies in and you shake them all about. **You do the hokey pokey to turn diabetes around.** That's what it's all about!

Did you know that **type-2 diabetes is reversible** for most people? It will take a little more than the hokey pokey to turn it around, but the movement helps too!

Staying sedentary can be absolutely detrimental to your health. Data from eight studies has shown that for every two hours people spend glued to the tube on a typical day, their risk of developing type-2 diabetes increases by 20% and their risk of heart disease increases by 15%.[10] If you can't miss your show, try hula-hooping or doing some yoga poses while watching!

Dr. Mark Hyman is a leading blood sugar expert and teacher at IIN. He believes that it is the very structure of our environment—Big Farming, Big Food, and Big Pharma, combined with the social, political, economic, and environmental conditions around us—that fosters and promotes the development of disease. In his book, *The Blood Sugar Solution*, he states, "It is how we eat, how much we exercise, how we manage stress, our exposure to environmental and food-based toxins, and the structural violence or 'obesogenic environment' that influences these factors are what is truly driving our Diabesity™ epidemic."

It's an epidemic—Americans are getting diabetes at an alarming rate! But those who are diagnosed often hold the power to cure themselves! Making healthy lifestyle changes to reduce obesity may reverse what has led to a type-2 diabetes diagnosis.

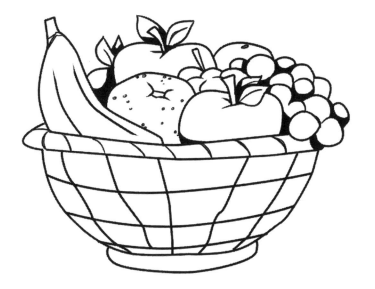

56

Secret

THESE LITTLE GUYS MAKE A BIG DIFFERENCE.

Getting enough of the following is really essential.

Antioxidants:

These are the powerful nutrients found in colorful fruits and vegetables. Each color represents beneficial properties our bodies needs to function at high levels. Practice eating a rainbow of colors everyday!

Vitamins:

These babies are needed to survive and thrive. Think vitality! There are fat-soluble vitamins that are stored in your fat to use over time, whereas water-soluble vitamins tend to flush out when you pee.

My favorite is folate—a type of B vitamin. There is plenty of folate in broccoli. I think of them as baby trees.

Minerals:

These are naturally occurring and are not manufactured by the body. We need larger amounts of essential minerals like calcium, potassium, and sodium, while we only need small amounts of others, such as iron, zinc, and magnesium.

The moral of this secret is to get you thinking about what your body needs and how to get it. **Eating a variety of local, seasonal fresh fruits and vegetables in all the different colors of the rainbow will most likely ensure you are getting what you need.**

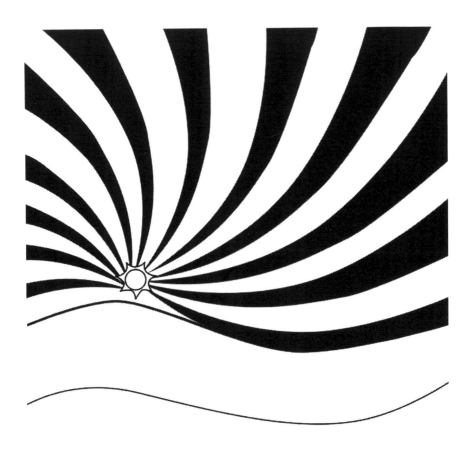

57

Secret

VITAMIN D = "VITAMIN DEFICIENT"

If you live north of Atlanta, chances are that you may be Vitamin D deficient from October through March!

Vitamin D is essential for calcium absorption, and deficiency is associated with bone pain and muscle weakness. When I started nutrition school I had major concerns about my vitamin D level. I decided to get tested after I graduated and believed I had improved my diet tremendously.

My vitamin D result was an 8.6, not even close to the minimum of 30-80 recommended by Western medicine. Holistic practitioners recommend that it be above 80 to prevent illnesses like heart disease and cancer.

A quick way to get a sense of your vitamin D levels is to place your thumb on your sternum. If it hurts, then you might have a vitamin D deficiency. Get tested by your doctor to find out for sure.

Get the information to make the necessary changes. Get lots of sunlight and healthy nutrition! **Work with your health care practitioner to bump up your levels if they are low.** But be aware that taking too much in supplemental form can be toxic.

I ended up needing to take 50,000 IU per week for three months to reach a level of 40.

I must tell you that I felt an amazing difference in my mind and body when my Vitamin D levels rose—my mood was also improved.

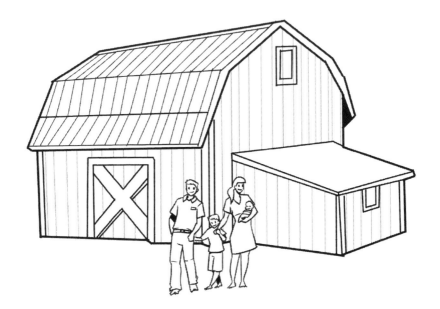

"Grow old along with me!
The best is yet to be..."

- Robert Browning

Vitamin B: Blessed Experiment— After cooking a meal, put a serving of food on two different plates. Place your hands in a prayer position and say a blessing of gratitude for one of the meals. Ask your friend or family member to choose a plate, and see which one they choose. Are they craving some of this special Vitamin B? Nine times out of ten they will choose the Blessed plate. **You have to try this.**

58

Secret

FINDING VITAMINS IN PLACES OTHER THAN FOOD.

Did you know that you can put energy into food, as well as getting energy from it?

Consider the different vitamins that are added to the foods you enjoy:

Vitamin L: Cooking with Love— Cooking with love is healthy! You will feel better after eating it. You will have better digestion and your body will be able to process all the nutrients.

Joshua Rosenthal calls Vitamin L the secret ingredient. To add extra love while you are cooking, practice by putting on dance tunes, smiling, singing, or doing whatever it takes to get that Vitamin L.

Vitamin H: Home Cooking— Are you noticing how much it costs you to eat out? Vitamin H is another term coined by Joshua Rosenthal. It stands for home-cooked meals. Home cooking not only saves you money, but it can be a much cleaner, healthier way to nourish you and your family.

Vitamin F: F-Bombs— Perhaps you can relate to this story. One day my friend ordered an almond bowl that took 10 minutes for the food preparer to assemble. As he was putting the finishing touches on the top, a banana came crashing down from the shelf above. The bowl tipped to the side and he immediately shouted the Vitamin F word!

Fortunately we were there to smile and lend support. Who would want all of that Vitamin F to go into the dish?! He was able to complete it with some Vitamin L. I know I've prepared some dishes with Vitamin F, haven't you? We can do better.

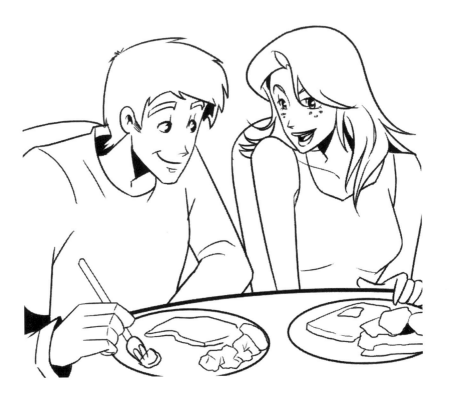

59

Secret

BE A FOODIE.

Foodies are game to try new things. I enjoyed being a "foodie" for a year and it was a wonderful experiment for my body. There were so many different flavors, textures, and foods that I didn't even know I was missing!

The idea is to buy a new food item that intrigues you every time you buy groceries. You'll be adding this one new food to your usual purchases. This way, if you don't like it, you'll still have your old stand-bys available.

If you do like it, you have something to add to your list of food "wins."

Are you wondering if this is even possible to do for a year? It is totally doable. Consider the variety of nuts, seeds, grains, vegetables, and fruits—the possibilities are endless!

Be a foodie for a year! Try a new food each week!

Keep life interesting!

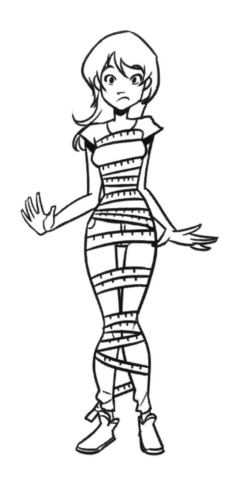

60

Secret

DIET IS ONE OF THE MOST OVERUSED WORDS IN NUTRITION.

Our culture is bombarded with the latest diet trends. Ask anyone, and they likely would agree!

While "diet" crazes have increased over the decades, we are seeing negative health effects increase with them. Furthermore, most of these diets have a huge failure rate, often because our bodies go into starvation mode and we end up storing fat!

Did you know that in 1992, Americans spent $30 billion on diet programs, pills, foods, and drinks? In 2007, we spent $55 billion. We now spend over $60 billion a year!

Wouldn't you think that all of this focus on dieting would change obesity rates for the better? Yet, in 1992, 12.6% of Americans were obese. Now 34.9% are obese.

Do you want out of this "diet" cycle? Me too!

Here's the simple solution: **Respect your body and eat real food.**

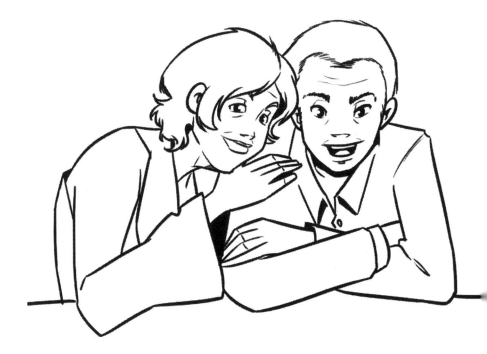

61

Secret

THE SKINNY ON OUR GRANDPARENTS.

What did your Grandma and Grandpa do every day when they were younger?

They walked, swept, vacuumed, mowed the lawn, washed the dishes, hung laundry, played with the kids... the list goes on and on.

They moved regularly every day! It was a way of life.

What about today? People lead sedentary lifestyles. They sit in front of electronics, they have others prepare their food and clean their homes, they drive instead of walk, and they hire specialists for nearly any service imaginable!

It's little wonder why some Americans are nearly 50 pounds heavier today.

Not so many decades ago, women averaged 110-115 pounds and men 150-165 pounds. They were in great shape!

Do you want to change the shape of your body?

Move like your grandparents did and while you are at it, eat like they did too!

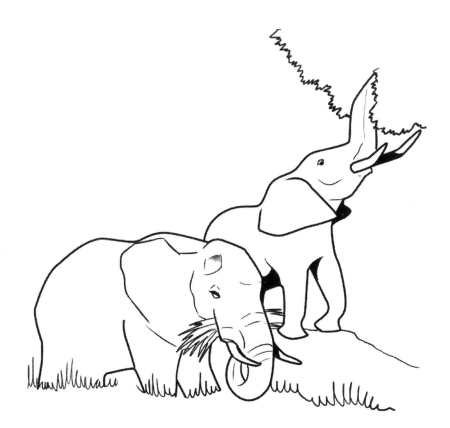

62

Secret

EAT LIKE AN ELEPHANT FOR STRONG BONES.

Elephants weigh 15,000 pounds on average and they live for 60 to 70 years. Those are some hefty numbers!

How do you think elephants support their enormous bodies? How do their bones stay healthy and strong?

It's through their diet and exercise of course! Elephants eat plenty of vegetables, especially leafy greens. This is where they get their calcium. These foods are also great for humans to get their calcium needs.

But what about calcium from milk, you ask? You won't need to drink milk if you get your calcium from other food sources.

How do you keep your bones strong in order to prevent osteoporosis and bone fractures?

According to John Robbins, author of *Diet for a New America,* "world health statistics show that osteoporosis is most common in exactly those countries where dairy products are consumed in the largest quantities—the United States, Finland, Sweden and the United Kingdom."

If you want to strengthen your bones, then eat like an elephant!

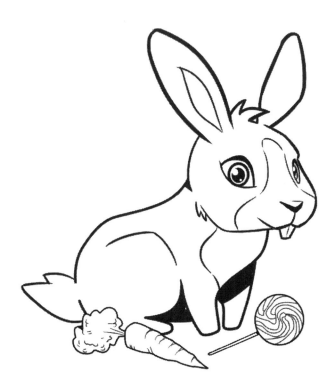

63

Secret

YOU'RE NOBODY UNTIL SOMEBUNNY LOVES YOU.

Chef Peter Evans shared a touching story (in his great Australian accent) about how he explained to his children why they should eat healthy food.

He knew how much they loved their pet bunny, and he wanted them to relate. He said, "**If I told you that your bunny would get weak and sick if we fed it lollies and pop,** would you want to feed it those foods?" They shook their heads no.

He continued, "What if I told you that **feeding your bunny veggies like carrots and celery would mean that your bunny would live a happy and healthy life**. Would you want to feed your bunny those foods?" His kids said yes.

Then he said, "Well you are my bunnies and I need to take care of you just like you want to take care of your bunny."

Such a simple and beautiful visual message.

Share it with the children you love!

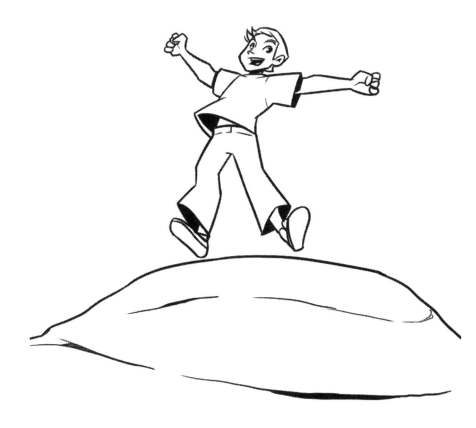

64

Secret

HOOKED ON A FEELING, HIGH ON BELIEVING...

Could craving something sweet have another meaning?

It might signify that you are craving a deeper connection with someone or something. The next time you reach for a pint of ice cream, ask yourself, "What are you really hungry for?" The answer might just surprise you!

Here are some reasons for cravings:

- **Toxic relationships**
- **Lack of water**
- **Food imbalance**
- **Lack of nutrients**
- **Hormonal**
- **Emotional**

Sweets can provide a temporary hormonal boost that imitates feelings of happiness. But the key word is temporary, and we are often left feeling worse because of the binge.

Check in with yourself to see what you might be craving and why. You might just need to give your body what it needs.

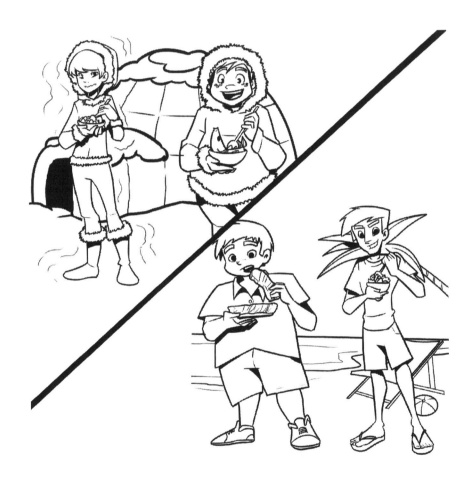

65

Secret

SKIP THE WHALE BLUBBER IN THE BAHAMAS.

Resources and foods will vary depending upon what part of the world you live in and the time of year—therefore your needs will vary too.

Regional foods provide additional nutrients and bacteria to sustain their local inhabitants. Do you take the time to consider how your region influences your food choices?

You wouldn't suggest that an Eskimo eat fresh fruits and citrus to stay warm all winter, would you? They would get too cold.

How about telling natives of the Bahamas to snack on some whale blubber in 100-degree heat? They'd probably die of a heart attack.

If it's winter and you're feeling cold, that's the time to add the healthy fats to keep warm. Conversely, if you are feeling hot this summer, that's when to turn toward to cooling fruits and vegetables.

Come on, do you really think people eat whale blubber in the Bahamas?

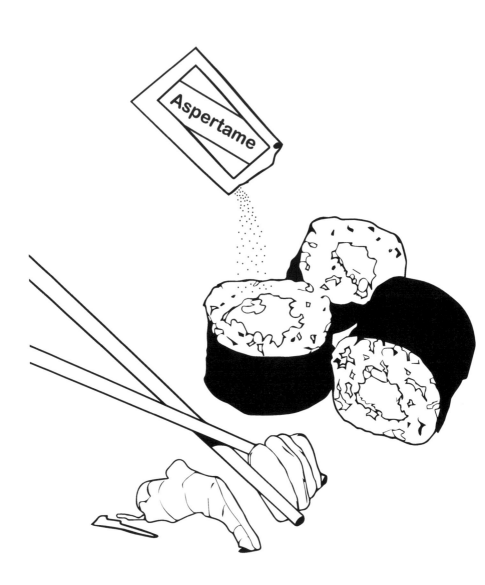

66

Secret

STICK TO THE UNSWEETENED SUSHI.

I was worried about the fish. I was surprised to find out I had to worry about the ginger, too.

Once, I went out to celebrate a friend's birthday at a highly rated Japanese restaurant, and one of the dishes had pink ginger on it.

I asked the chef if it was prepared fresh or served from a package. His response left me dumbfounded! It was packaged with the artificial sweetener aspartame and contained food dye.

When I inquired further, he told me it was the second ingredient after the ginger. When I mentioned that I was "sensitive" to artificial sweeteners, he offered to make me a new dish. I gladly accepted!

Always think about what's in your food. Even a fancy restaurant could be using artificial coloring and sweeteners.

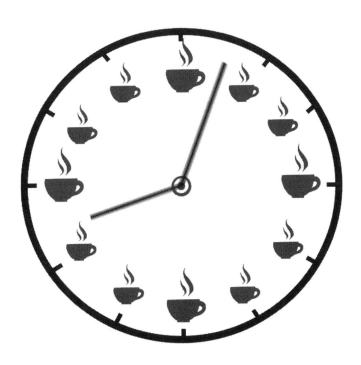

67

Secret

COFFEE ISN'T JUST FOR BREAKFAST ANYMORE.

Coffee is a widely used drug of choice!

During my experience at nutrition school, I decided that it was time to quit caffeine and lessen the anxiety it caused. In order to kick my addiction, I was advised to remove it slowly from my diet.

First I started with:

- Week 1: ¾ of a cup regular and ¼ decaf

- Week 2: ½ cup of regular and ½ decaf

- Week 3: ¼ cup regular and ¾ decaf

- Week 4: Finally, full decaf with just a splash of regular

- Week 5: Off caffeine!

Even when you wean yourself off of caffeine slowly, you may experience withdrawal symptoms. Drink lots of water and find a fun replacement drink. **To release some of the emotional and physical symptoms, keep a bag of coffee around to "sniff"** if needed. If you love the coffee aroma, don't deprive yourself.

If you aren't ready to give up the coffee, consider switching to a healthier, less-caffeinated version! Organic, fair-trade, shaded espresso beans brewed as coffee is my favorite!

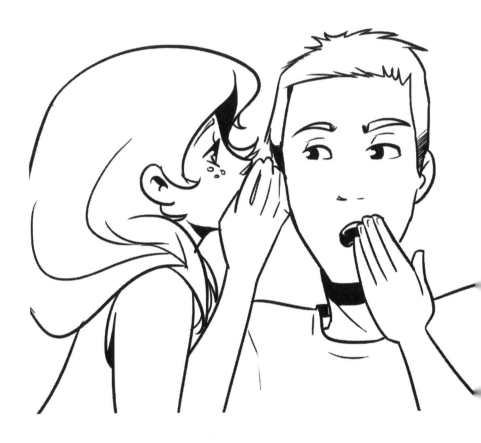

68

Secret

YOU'RE NOT SICK; YOU'RE THIRSTY.

Do you have a headache? Are you feeling droopy, foggy, or slow? How do you bring yourself back up to par?

Have you seen how easily **your plants revive when you give them some much-needed water**? Imagine what water can do for you.

"Don't treat thirst with medication," says Dr. F. Batmanghelidj, "chronic dehydration contributes to and even produces pain and many degenerative diseases that can be prevented and treated by increasing water intake on a regular basis."

Sometimes the answer is simpler than you think. Grab a glass of refreshing spring water. If you have signs of dehydration (such as thirst, tiredness, dark urine, headache, and dry skin) you need to replenish yourself.

A good rule of thumb is to drink half of your body weight (in ounces) of water every day. If you weigh 120 pounds, practice drinking 60 ounces a day. That is only about 7 to 8 cups.

Drink up before you go searching through the medicine cabinet or rushing to the local pharmacy!

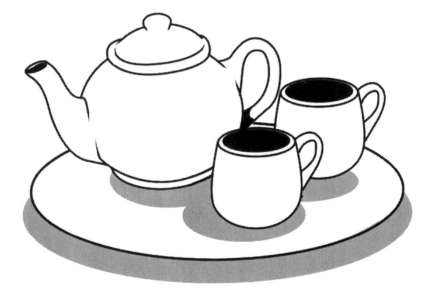

69

Secret

DRINKING BOILING WATER IS GOOD TO THE LAST DROP!

Did you know that you can sip your way back to healthy digestion?

Try this easy Ayurvedic practice. First, boil some water. Then take a sip of it every 10 minutes. See if you can do this during the day for two weeks.

I tried this and after a few days, I was hooked! My incredible results included feeling more hydrated and less groggy. I also felt like I had a flatter tummy.

Dr. John Douillard, director of LifeSpa Ayurvedic Center, explains that boiled water loosens the heavy minerals that have caused disruption in the digestive tract. An additional bonus is that it flushes out your lymphatic system, which is like a drainage system for the body.

At end of the experiment, if you're still feeling thirsty, it may mean that you were more dehydrated than you realized!

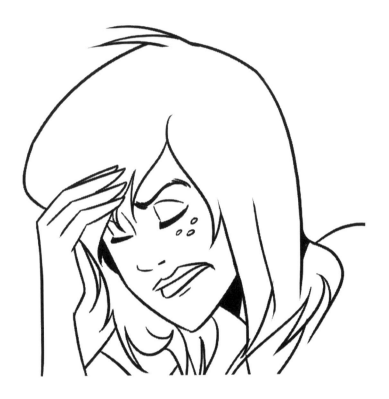

I had the honor of meeting Dr. Annemarie Colbin at a Friday night dinner at NGI. I shared my headache issues with her and she said, "Dear, you are having liver headaches." Ever since that time I have been better able to prevent and manage any headaches that arise and they rarely become migraines now.

Additional headache secrets — headaches can also result from **hormonal changes**. These require getting the body back into balance. Remember to keep **hydrated** as mentioned earlier in Secret #68. If you continue to suffer from headaches or migraines, make sure to speak to your doctor so you can rule out more serious issues.

If you are suffering from headaches due to **environmental, food or seasonal allergies** it is time to clean out your body and home.

For **hangover** headaches remember our miracle juice combination in Secret #31 and get some sleep.

70

Secret

IT'S TIME TO LET YOUR HEADACHES GO.

I used to suffer from weekly headaches and migraines. This resulted in many hours of missed work, time with friends, special occasions, and living with a terrible quality of life.

Dr. Annemarie Colbin, Founder of The Natural Gourmet Institute for Health and Culinary Arts (NGI) in New York City was a guest speaker at nutrition school, and I devoured her lecture about migraines and headaches. She taught us about these **5 different types of headaches and how to prevent them.**

1) **Expansive** — suffering from eating too many sweet foods. REMEDY: Balance that by eating salty foods like olives or umeboshi plums.

2) **Contractive** — suffering from eating too many salty foods. REMEDY: Eat sweet foods like applesauce, organic frozen fruit bars or juices. Drink plenty of water too!

3) **Liver** — usually occur about 3 hours after consuming too much fat on an empty stomach. REMEDY: You need lemon! Keep lemon popsicles, lemons and lemon juice around at all times—especially if you suffer from migraines. Make lemon tea with the juice of ½ lemon. Then, boil the remaining peel and pulp in 1 1/4 c. water for about 10 minutes. Add to the juice and drink.

4) **Caffeine** — caused by reducing or cutting out caffeine too quickly. REMEDY: Immediately have some caffeine or follow Secret #67 to reduce it slowly over time.

5) **Structural** — suffering from misalignment or injury. REMEDY: See a physical therapist or chiropractor to get you back on track.

Practice being mindful by keeping a journal of your daily food intake and routine to evaluate if one of these remedies may work for you.

Attending IIN was worth it for this reason alone. I love to share this secret!

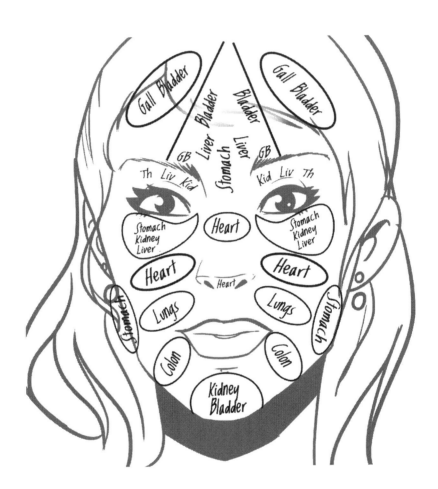

71

Secret

FACE IT, YOUR ORGANS ARE TALKING TO YOU.

A little information goes a long way. **Just look at this map and compare it to the any bumps on your face.**

Recently, I started having breakouts around my eyebrows. I was actually doing a liver cleanse. It all made sense. I could see that my body was actually showing me signals of what was going on in my body!

While working on a client, I couldn't get over how many zits and bumps she had around her nose. I decided to pull out my chart and found that the bumps there indicated that it was related to her heart. I gently suggested that she go to the doctor and get her blood pressure checked. We were both glad she did because it was 180 over 138, way too high! Danger zone high!

Whether you are getting your period and seeing break outs on your chin, or have a strange bump in your ear, pay attention to what your organs are telling you.

I find it is always helpful to have a guide to help us get in touch with what is going on in our bodies!

Keep this chart handy and tell a friend!

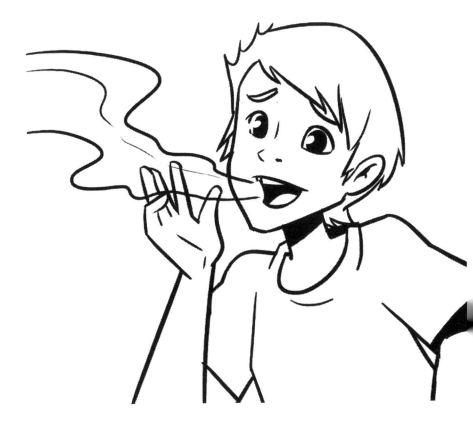

72

Secret

YOUR DENTAL HEALTH SAYS A LOT ABOUT YOU!

When is the last time you flossed? If you knew that it could save your life would you make time for it? My dentist told me it is the number one thing I can do for my heart.

Did you know that heart disease and oral health are linked?

Ever wonder what plaque is? It's that sticky film of bacteria on your teeth. People with periodontitis issues should know that chewing your food and tooth-brushing can release bacteria into the bloodstream. We don't want the plaque to end up in the arteries of your heart.

Don't "stress out"—just make sure you floss and brush your teeth regularly. Your heart will thank you!

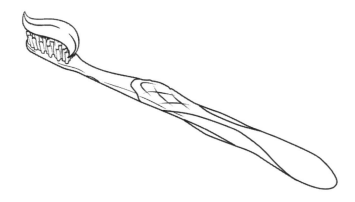

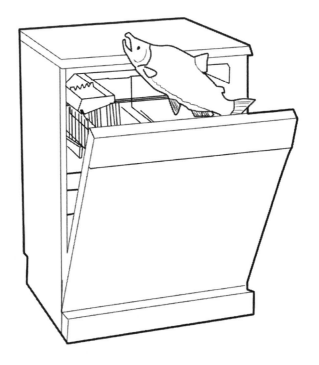

73

Secret

GET WILD AND COOK SALMON IN THE DISHWASHER!

Now that I have your attention... I just wanted to let you know it is okay to relax and make things fun in the kitchen. Think outside the box—and in the dishwasher!

Jammin' Dishwasher Salmon Recipe
by Dude Food (Serves 4)

- 2 pounds center cut salmon fillet (no thicker than 1-1/4 inches)
- 1 orange, cut into 1/8 inch slices
- 4 tablespoons orange juice concentrate
- 1 teaspoon fresh or dried thyme

1. Rinse the salmon fillet and pat dry. Remove any noticeable bones with needle nose pliers.

2. On a flat surface, pull out a length of aluminum foil long enough to cover and fold over the fish, plus a little extra. Place the orange slices in the middle and arrange the salmon on top. Spread the concentrate over the salmon and sprinkle with the thyme. Bring the short ends of the foil together, meeting in the middle of the fish. Align the edges evenly and fold them over at least twice, crimping the final edge. Bring the long sides together, folding and crimping in the same manner.

3. Place the bundle on the top rack of an empty dishwasher. Close the door and set the machine on a normal cycle. When the cycle is completed, remove the salmon – it should be moist and cooked through. If not, run back through the cycle another 5 to 7 minutes. Unwrap and transfer to a serving platter.

Okay, so I didn't try this recipe because I actually use my dishwasher for storage but I hope to make this one day!

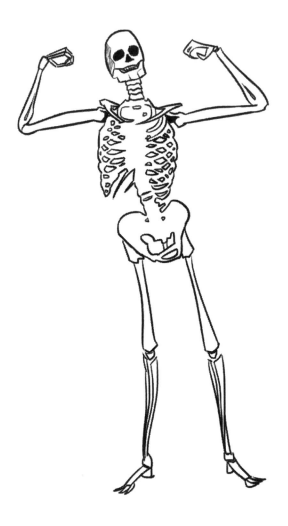

74

Secret

MILK CAN ACTUALLY DO A BODY BRITTLE.

Milk is tricky these days, even the non-dairy kind.

Animal milk is intended to nurture its own species. Cow's milk is intended to feed calves which eventually grow to be 400 pounds. If you want to be 400 pounds, then drinking cow's milk to excess is the way to go!

For reasons not yet fully understood, countries with the highest intake of dairy also have the highest rates of osteoporosis.

Human beings are the only animal that consumes dairy after weaning with milk from another species.

For these reasons, consuming dairy could be considered "unnatural." Hunter-gatherers didn't drink milk after weaning. They got calcium from many other sources. This demonstrates that dairy is unnecessary from an evolutionary perspective.

The nutritional theories and studies on dairy are abundant and frequently changing, and I encourage you to go deeper and explore this for yourself. If you can't give up your dairy, AT LEAST be sure to buy organic!

There are great dairy-free alternatives on the market. Here are some of my favorites: **Coconut milk, Almond milk, Rice milk, Cashew milk, Hemp milk.**

Avoid: Any milks with the preservative carrageenan, added flavors, and sugars. Soy milk has been highly controversial because it is most likely genetically modified (and may alter estrogen levels), therefore should be avoided.

So where will your calcium come from? **Remember from Secret #62 that elephants love their greens!**

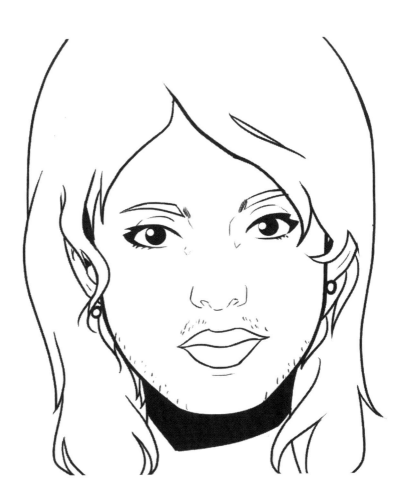

75

Secret

SUGAR IS A HAIRY PROBLEM.

As an electrologist, I've seen over a thousand cases of women with **excessive body hair, many of whom suffer from polycystic ovarian syndrome** (PCOS).

PCOS is one of the most common hormonal disorders in women. Many women with **PCOS suffer from insulin resistance, type-2 diabetes, high cholesterol, high blood pressure, and heart disease.** Most often they suffer from **excessive facial and body hair, depression, heavy periods, and obesity.**

By far, the biggest lifestyle contributor to PCOS is poor diet. Young women with PCOS tend to eat far too much sugar and highly refined carbohydrates. Not only does sugar spike insulin levels, but it also contributes to high blood pressure and an increased risk of heart disease in women with PCOS. The unhealthy rise in insulin levels wreaks havoc with the hormones that are responsible for causing most PCOS symptoms.

It is a very difficult disease to diagnose and treat. However, I have seen many women change their lives by cleaning up their diets and getting their hormones back in balance. Also, increasing their vitamin D exposure and other key nutritional aspects seem to be very effective.

If you are suffering from hormonal issues or PCOS, remember you can do something about it!

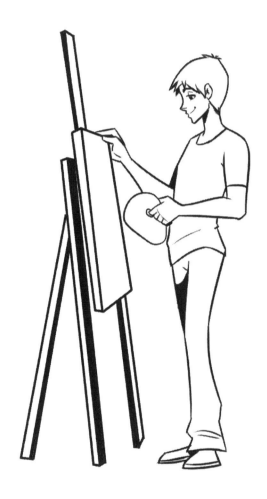

76

Secret

GET OUT THE ART SUPPLIES.

Have you ever enjoyed coloring with a child? Relaxing and fulfilling, isn't it? Drawing can be therapeutic, which is why many mental health treatments often include art therapy.

Did you know that it can be used to improve physical health too?

Bernie Siegel is a renowned expert in cancer care. He's a physician who also works to strengthen the immune system through the mind-body connection.

In his latest book, *The Art of Healing: Uncovering Your Inner Wisdom and Potential for Self-Healing,* Dr. Siegel explains that **the use of drawing in his practice has helped patients discover the physical, psychological, and emotional aspects of healing and guided them toward the best choices and options for their particular situation.**

Why? Drawing often produces symbols representing the subconscious. Dr. Siegel shows how **to interpret drawings to help with everything from understanding why we are sick to making treatment decisions and communicating with loved ones.**

He asserts that no matter your artistic background, you can learn a lot about yourself and your health by drawing pictures.

So what is your art telling you? How is it making you feel?

Please, go find out! Find a "paint night" near you!

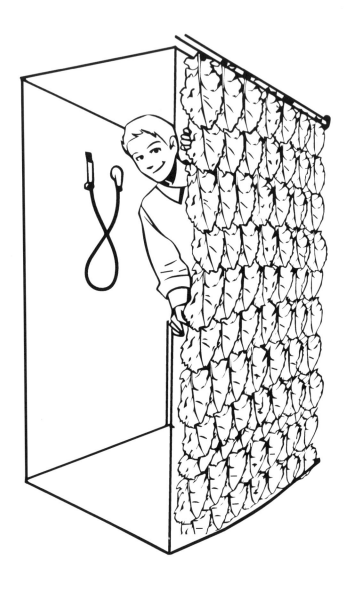

77

Secret

DON'T HIDE BEHIND THE KALE CURTAIN.

You know those people who live behind the "Kale Curtain," the ones thinking that they are living a healthy lifestyle just because they eat the right foods?

The truth is, it doesn't matter how much kale or healthy food you eat if your life is out of balance or if you surround yourself with people who are toxic.

Even a gluten-free, vegan, yoga addict can get sick if the Primary Food areas are toxic.

That girl next to you at the gym snacking on kale could hate her job, boyfriend and be bankrupt.

Evaluate the toxic people and things in your life. Notice how much time you are spending with them. Shift your energy and your health can change. You need to eat right and live the good life too!

But I must admit—eating kale is still a really wise choice.

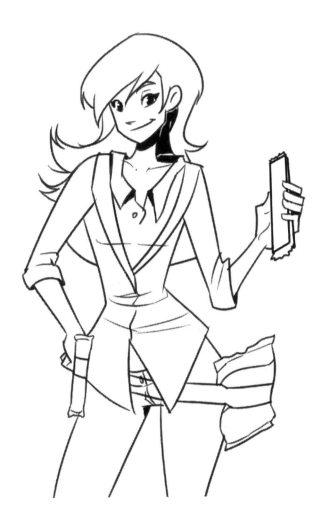

78

Secret

YOUR MOOD CAN GO STRAIGHT TO YOUR HIPS LIKE A BAG OF CHIPS.

Let's get this straight. Our moods affect us.

Ever wonder what feeds your emotions? Your food and mood go hand in hand.

Our mood greatly affects the food choices we make. The Food Mood Girl and fellow health coach, Lindsey Smith, shares some of her wisdom.

"My recipe to health and happiness and to food and mood balancing is to, 'Think Good Thoughts, Eat Real Food, Love Yourself, and Repeat as Necessary.' I think we need all elements to truly find a good balance in our food and mood relationship. Recognizing that what we eat affects how we feel is the first step. Most times when we eat crap, we feel like crap. Or if we feel like crap, we want to eat crap. Nourishing your body and loving yourself fully are two things that can help boost your mood and make it a sustainable lifestyle."

What you eat affects your mood and not just immediately. Sometimes it takes one, two, or three days for your body to digest your food. Pay attention to what you eat and how you feel a few hours later to a few days later. Once you start seeing patterns and making connections, you can truly heal your mood.

Every step away from the chips is a great step towards better health.

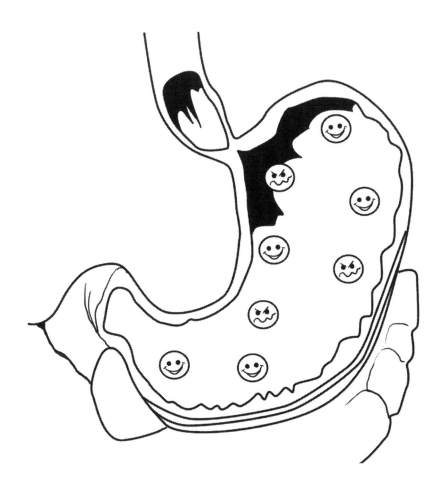

"All disease starts with candida."

—Donna Gates

79

Secret

CHECK IN WITH YOUR GUT!

Everyone has bacteria in their tummies to break down food and keep their immune system balanced. Think of your body as having its own eco system that needs to be in balance to prevent illness.

Many of my clients have suffered from frequent yeast and bacterial infections. Often their doctors would prescribe antibiotics to kill off the bacterial infections which can lead to a new problem: candida—an overgrowth of yeast.

When Donna Gates, gut health expert and author of the *Body Ecology Diet*, appeared as a guest speaker at one of our nutrition conferences, I was very interested in what she would say about yeast infections and the suggested remedies.

The most shocking thing I learned was her belief that candidiasis —a systemic yeast infection, has become a silent pandemic.

She went on to explain:

- All children with **autism** test positive for yeast in the gut.
- **Alzheimer's** patients have yeast infections that interfere with neurotransmitters in the brain.
- **Asthma** sufferers have yeast in the lungs.
- All those with **Fibromyalgia** have systemic yeast overgrowth.

To clear out excess yeast and fungi from the body she recommends:

- Raising physical energy levels — ensuring proper rest.
- Conquering infection — starving the yeast that lives on sugar.
- Correcting digestion — Eating a diet high in nourishing plant and sea vegetables, probiotic foods, and taking enzymes.
- Safely cleaning out excess toxins from the body.

This powerful program has been shown to prevent and even cure many diseases. Donna Gates' visionary work needs to be spread like wildfire.

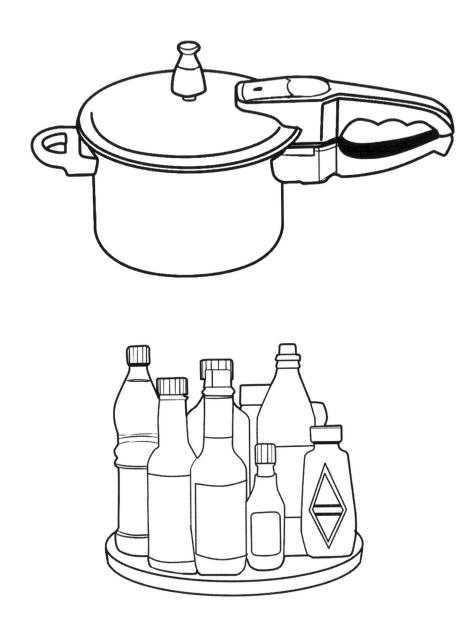

80

Secret

RELEASE THE STRESS AND JUST COOK UNDER PRESSURE.

These are my favorite time-saving kitchen tools to make your life super easy!

Pressure cooker: Makes for speedy cooking, flavorful dishes and the bonus of easy cleanup!

Salad spinner: Dries greens fast! No more soggy salads!

Meat thermometer: Critical to cooking meat to safe temperatures.

Garlic press: Let's face it—no one has time to properly dice cloves of garlic.

Grapefruit spoon: Can also be used for butternut squash, pumpkins, melons and papayas!

Lazy Susan: Spin the wheel of flavor

Need to spice up your meals? The lazy Susan is the perfect way to start exploring and making good use of your time. You can make boiled or broiled chicken in advance, without flavoring much. Then fill up your lazy Susan with different spices, condiments, and dressings so people can spice up their own chicken or meal themselves. This saves cooking time, is super fun, and gives people the opportunity to flavor to their unique taste. The kids can get into it, too!

Give these gadgets a go!

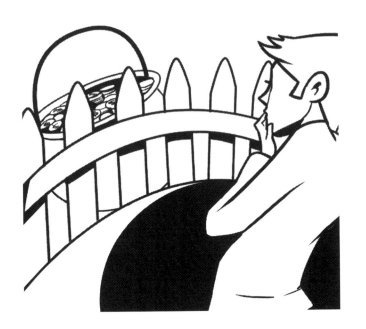

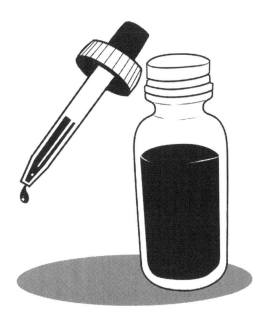

81

Secret

AN OUNCE OF PREVENTION IS A HEALTHY POT OF GOLD.

What can you do when everyone around you is sick and you want to avoid catching a cold or flu? **Hydrate and lubricate!**

Hot water and lemon isn't just for grandma—it's the best tonic available year-round. **Warm lemon water can help cleanse your body, keep you hydrated, and give your body a boost of nutrients**. Lemon water helps flush out toxins, balances your pH level, and helps reduce the symptoms of the common cold.

Drink this tonic first thing in the morning to help your body prepare for the day. If you feel a cold coming on, drink lemon water throughout the day to help kick the cold for good. For an extra boost **add cayenne pepper to soothe coughs and sore throats. It has also been shown to break up mucus.**

To keep your sinuses lubricated try this: once a week, put a little warmed oil (olive oil and garlic) in your ears before bed. Use an eye dropper or tincture dropper to place a few drops of body temperature oil in the ears.

Mark Hyman, a Functional Medicine doctor, also suggests doing a daily nasal saline flush, eating lots of garlic, onions, and ginger and of course getting lots of sleep!

There you go—your pot of gold.

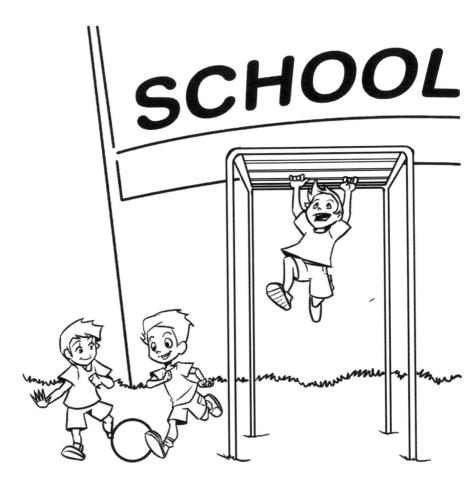

82

Secret

RECESS OVER RITALIN.

ADHD is certainly a hot topic these days. There is lots of evidence on all sides. Let's go deeper.

In discussing the benefits of physical activity on children's behavior, internationally renowned expert in nutrition, as well as guest speaker at IIN, David Katz, asserted, "Recess, not Ritalin." I couldn't agree more!

He states that rates of behavioral disorders in childhood—attention deficit disorder in particular—are at an all-time high. Why is that? **Children are much the same as they ever were. But their typical day has changed drastically.** Kids used to walk to school, do chores around the house, and play physical games for entertainment (rather than electronic ones). Frustratingly, school systems are feeling a budget crunch, so are looking for ways to cut costs. Oftentimes, it's the arts and enrichment classes, physical education, recess, and organized sports that get cut out of our children's day.

Dr. Olga Jarrett, with her colleagues at Georgia State University's Department of Early Childhood Education, observed two fourth-grade classes in an urban school with a strict no-recess policy. They implemented recess once a week so they could observe the children's behavior on recess and non-recess days. Their results showed that the 43 children became more on-task and less fidgety on days when they had recess. Sixty percent of the children, including five with attention deficit disorder, worked more and/or fidgeted less on recess days.

Kids need to be kids. They need to explore, climb, jump, run around, and play. Bring back recess!

Note: I do not wish to hurt or judge those who use medications. Each individual must decide with a doctor what is right for their situation or condition, and what course of action is right for them or their child.

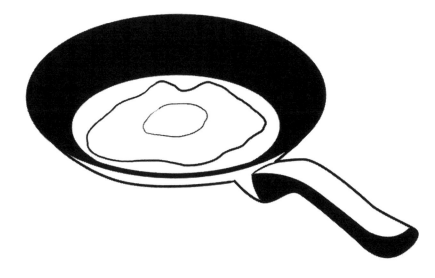

83
Secret

TURN YOUR DAY SUNNY SIDE UP.

Eggs are considered by many to be nature's perfect food.

They are loaded with protein, vitamins, and minerals, as well as important fatty acids that help the brain and nervous system remain sharp.

Contrary to what we have been taught for many years, eating **more** eggs actually doesn't have a negative effect on heart disease.

Remember; don't skip the yolk because incredible nutrition is packed in there. It contains vitamin B12, choline, and biotin, and it's also rich in anti-oxidants like lutein and, yup, cholesterol. Despite the fact that cholesterol has been given a bad name, it is important for hormone function, and it's a component of every single cell in our bodies.

My personal favorite—local, farm-fresh and free-range eggs. They taste so much better than store-bought factory-farmed eggs... try them!

Life is great over-easy too!

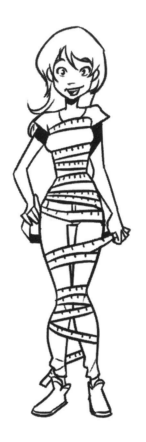

Take off the tape!

84

Secret

DON'T BE AFRAID TO LIVE A LITTLE.

When I began my journey at IIN I was completely excited to be trying all kinds of new foods to learn about the often conflicting information and nutritional theories. After a few months my head was spinning. Was there anything safe enough to eat?

Healthy eating, like anything else, can be unhealthy when taken to the extreme. In fact, there is a term for it—orthorexia nervosa—first coined by Steven Bratman, MD, in his book *Health Food Junkies*. It involves obsession with eating only foods that are personally acceptable in terms of health, calories, or origin and it causes anxiety, ritualistic thoughts and behaviors, and excessive pickiness with food. Orthorexia nervosa is a serious mental condition that can impair your life and daily functioning.

Women's leadership coach and fellow IIN graduate Nisha Moodley says that at one point she was terrified to eat food that didn't fit within her framework of what was healthy. She was terrified she would get cancer and die.

I was less overwhelmed when I started to figure out that there were many foods that worked for my mind and body. **We need to develop healthy eating preferences, instead of obsessions, and get beyond labeling food as good and bad.**

You don't have to strive for perfection—remember the 80/20 rule. Food is meant to be enjoyed!

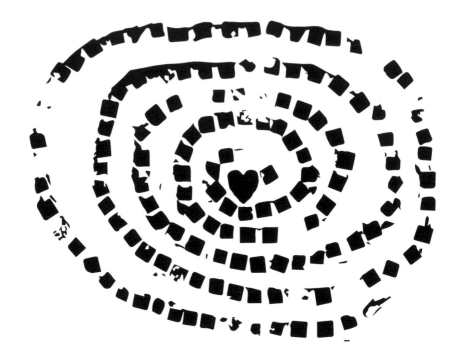

Special Artist:

Lexington Anthony

Be yourself and truly use your own words.

Your words are your truth—they are your wisdom.
They are your power.

Do your best, be unique, and keep moving forward on your journey

If you always put your heart into it the first time you will
be living a life with no regrets.

85

Secret

PUT YOUR HEART INTO IT THE FIRST TIME.

Your word is one of the most important aspects of your character that you have to share with the world. If you say something, you should mean it!

Being authentic and living your truth is just as important for your health as what you put on your plate.

One of my favorite IIN instructors and mentor, Marilena Minucci said this, **"Your authenticity comes from having learned from, transformed, and transcended your 'story'... not from living it over and over again."**

It is so important to forgive yourself for the past to free up your energy to live in a more heart-centered way, honoring and accepting yourself.

Living this way will improve your inward and outward communication, and will minimize any guessing, assumptions, and half-truths. Many of us believe that little white lies are okay, but if you make the commitment to honor your integrity, even the slightest divergence from the truth won't feel good in your body.

If you are noticing that you are stretching a 'story' in any area of your life, drop the story. You will be able to deal with situations when you are clear with yourself and others about what is going on.

You may begin to notice that your relationships will strengthen— from your loved ones to your bill collectors—when you do what you say and say what you mean!

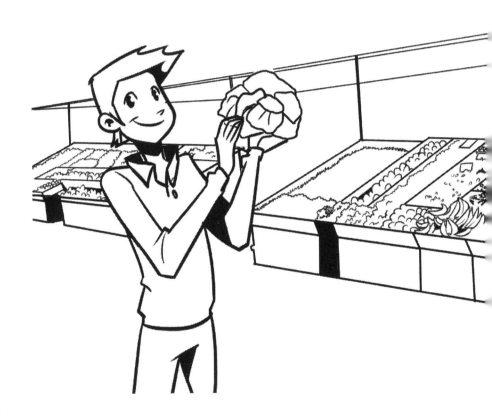

86

Secret

STOP SPENDING TOO MUCH MONEY ON SUPPLEMENTS.

How many supplement bottles are cluttering your medicine cabinet? Adding to your grocery bills?

I remember Dr. Andrew Weil asking us—if we were going to live on a deserted island, what items would we take with us, INCLUDING our supplements? The crowd erupted in giggles.

Up to half of all adults in the United States take a multivitamin. Most probably expect it to make them feel better and prevent common illnesses, even though the evidence has always been a little sketchy. Is your daily multivitamin habit truly effective—or just wishful thinking?

Nothing can surpass the amazing benefits of eating whole fruits and vegetables packed with amazing antioxidants, vitamins and nutrients as well as with other minerals and biological factors that help with absorption and digestion.

I only recommend that my clients take supplements if they've been found to be deficient or fighting some type of illness. In those cases, it is important to make sure they are getting reliable, quality, safe products—and that they don't take them for long periods of time.

Whatever money you are spending on your supplements, it's probably better to spend it at the farmer's market or the grocery store on healthy whole foods.

I have tried to stop browsing too!

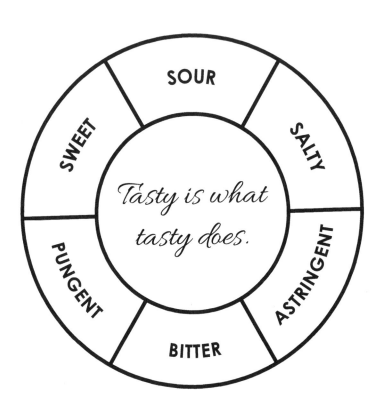

87

Secret

TAKE TIME FOR TASTY!

The practice of Ayurveda teaches that all six tastes should be eaten at every meal for us to feel satisfied and to ensure that all major food groups and nutrients are represented.

1. **Sweet** foods are made of carbs, protein, and fat, and include grains, starchy vegetables, dairy, meat, chicken, fish, sugar, honey, and molasses. They have a soothing effect on the body, bring about satisfaction, and build body mass.

2. **Sour** foods contain organic acids and include citrus, berries, tomatoes, pickled foods, salad dressing, and alcohol. They stimulate the appetite and aid digestion (but can be irritating to those who suffer from heartburn).

3. **Salty** foods contain mineral salts and include table salt, soy sauce, salted meats, and fish. They enhance the appetite and make other tastes more delicious.

4. **Pungent** foods contain essential oils and include peppers, chilies, onions, garlic, cayenne, black pepper, cloves, ginger, mustard, and salsa. They promote sweating and clear the sinus passages.

5. **Bitter** foods contain alkaloids or glycosides, and include green leafy vegetables, green and yellow vegetables, kale, celery, broccoli, sprouts, and beets. These foods detoxify the system, but may cause some gas or indigestion.

6. **Astringent** foods contain tannins and include lentils, dried beans, green apples, grape skins, cauliflower, pomegranates, and tea.

Have fun and explore those taste buds!

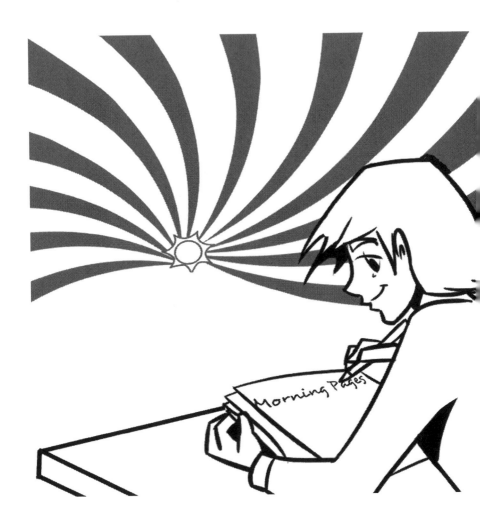

88

Secret

ALL GOOD THINGS COME TO THOSE WHO WRITE THEIR MORNING PAGES.

One of the most life-changing lessons in nutrition school was completing the morning pages activity by Julia Cameron, author of *The Artist's Way*.

Exploring creativity and writing in nutrition school seems a bit odd, but honestly, it completely changed my health.

Being creative sets the tone for health, happiness, and success. Waking up early and writing out your thoughts can spark many insights, creative processes, and changes you want to make in all areas of your life. I was surprised to find that my to-do list for the day, my goals list, as well as my deepest feelings and thoughts found their way into the morning pages. It is that powerful.

Now it's your turn, let's see what you can create!

Wake up 20 minutes early—so you are still in that state just before complete wakefulness. Write three pages long hand (not typed). Just write whatever comes to your mind, don't edit. The exercise is not meant to be perfect.

Personally, I feel more "alive" doing the morning pages. It starts my day on such a deep spiritual level that I feel like I am on cloud nine for the entire day.

The very idea for writing this book came from morning pages. Try it!

I feel comfortable throwing out a guarantee your life will change!

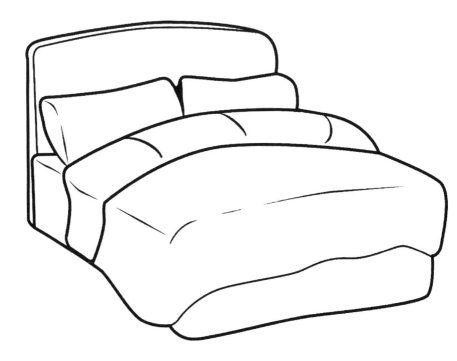

"With sleep and proper rest—everything is transformed.
Sleep deprivation should no longer be a badge of honor."

— Arianna Huffington

Creator of the Huffington Post and Author of *Thrive*

89
Secret

SLEEP IS THE NEW WONDER DRUG.

Did I just give you permission to use a drug?

Sure, we know sleep is important for us, yet we tend to deny ourselves.

Scientists have discovered that sleep is not just important for the brain, but also for immune function, hormone balancing, learning, and my favorite, weight loss.

Sleep is the time when your body repairs all the damage done to it during the day.

Sleep deprivation can increase your risk of high blood pressure, diabetes, depression, obesity, and cancer.

I live in the city that never sleeps: New York City. Here, sleep is not a valued commodity. It's almost unheard of for people to put in less than a 12-hour workday, and nearly all of us bring work home.

When people don't get enough sleep they aren't as productive. Not to mention, they are more irritable and prone to short tempers that are often disruptive and embarrassing.

So go ahead, try it. Shut off your phone. Fall into bed. Wrap yourself in a blanket. And deeply inhale the freedom of giving your body exactly what it needs... a good night's sleep.

Sweet Dreams!

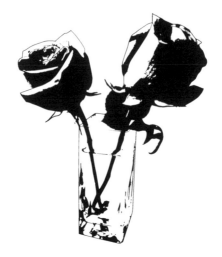

WEALTH & PROSPERITY	FAME & REPUTATION	LOVE & MARRIAGE
Persistent Wind	Clinging Fire	Recaptive Earth
Rear left, blues, purple & reds	Rear middle *Fire* Reds	Red Right Reds, Pinks & whites
WEALTH & FAMILY	**CENTER HEALTH**	**CREATIVITY & CHILDREN**
Shocking Thunder		Joyous lake
Middle left *Wood* Blues & greens	Center *Earth* Yellow/earthtones	Middle Right *Metal* White & pastels
KNOWLEDGE & SELF-CULTIVATION	**CAREER**	**HELPFUL PEOPLE & TRAVEL**
Still Mountain	Deep Water	Heaven
Front Left Black,blues & green	Front Middle *Water* Black & Dark middle tones	Front Right White, grays & black

Notice that heath
is at the center of it all.

90

Secret

CREATE YOUR SPACE.

Translated, feng shui means "air and water" in Chinese. It means that you can make sense of peace in your space.

Kate Mackinnon, one of my teachers at IIN gave a beautiful lecture on Feng Shui. Our assignment was to close our eyes and go to a special place in your mind—describe what you see around you.

Almost all people will describe a special place in nature. What you see around you means something to you whether it is warmth, safety, abundance, or love.

The purpose of feng shui is to bring positive energy into your life, and the best place to start is the home. If you are interested in this ancient practice and want to learn more, you might consider bringing a specialist into your home to create your purposeful, loving space that will help you accomplish your goals, usually regarding love, money, power, and health.

We should all be inspired to make our living spaces clean, livable and user friendly. Imagine if your home and office were a peaceful place to be!

My favorite tip for those **looking for love**: place two rosebuds in a vase next to your bed. When they die, discard and replace them. I hope you will just love the way they look, smell and the added benefit of realizing that you are taking time to do something loving for yourself. You may just find that more love may want to enter the room too.

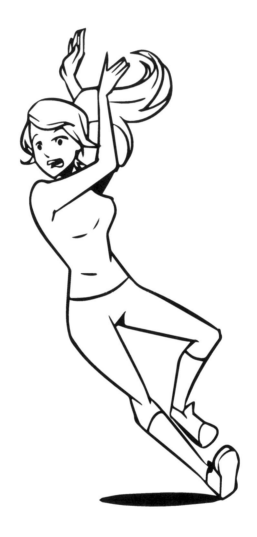

Stumbling is your early detection signal.

91

Secret

STUMBLING IS THE SIGNAL TO SLOW DOWN.

Falling out of your Tree Pose? Your Downward Dog feeling a bit stiff? Have you found yourself stumbling quite a bit lately?

Take notice. It is time to slow down. It's a good time to step back and get our bodies and minds back in check. Listening to our bodies is key to staying happy and healthy.

Your body is constantly seeking balance. When we notice that "everything feels off," it probably is.

Check in and think about your recent eating patterns and how life in general is going. If you are eating a ton of salty foods, your body may start craving something sweet. If you are sad, take a second to see what is happening in your body. Do you feel stiff? Need a cry? Or are you craving a cookie? This is the natural human tendency. **If you ever feel out of balance, see what you need more of in order to get back on track.**

After you take some time for yourself and rebalance you will be able get moving again.

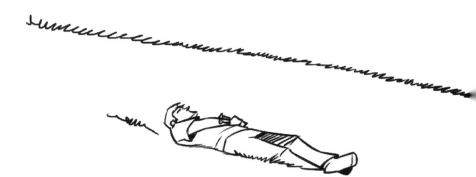

Practice this one last meditation.

Lie down, close your eyes, imagine that your cares and worries are in the clouds—and ALLOW them to pass by. This too shall pass.

92

Secret

MEDITATION CHANGES EVERYTHING.

Most of us lead very busy lives, and finding the time to turn inward and meditate each day can be a struggle. Meditation allows us to collect our thoughts, recover our strength, and to see things in a fresh perspective.

Meditation is simply a method of training the mind to become peaceful. When our minds are quiet, we free ourselves from worries and mental discomfort, and we allow true happiness to arise.

Meditation can also help with physical ailments—you can visualize your way to health and comfort. Practice this: **Take a deep breath, imagining brilliant white light traveling down to whatever pain or illness you may have.** Hold the breath in that area and imagine the light engulfing all your pain or illness. When it is time to exhale, release your pain in a cloud of black smoke and visualize the toxins that are leaving your body forever. Repeat as needed.

I always imagined that meditation was "strange" until I experienced its positive effects by practicing these techniques presented by Thich Nhat Hanh, a Vietnamese Zen Buddhist monk, teacher, and author of *Peace is Every Step*.

These practices can transform your life; make an effort to try them.

1. When sitting at a **traffic light**—take the opportunity to find gratitude for something in your life.

2. When the **phones rings**—wait for the third ring and take a moment to center yourself before greeting the caller.

3. When **feeling alone**—give yourself a hug. Sometimes the adult in you needs to hug your inner child because you are the only one who can reach that place.

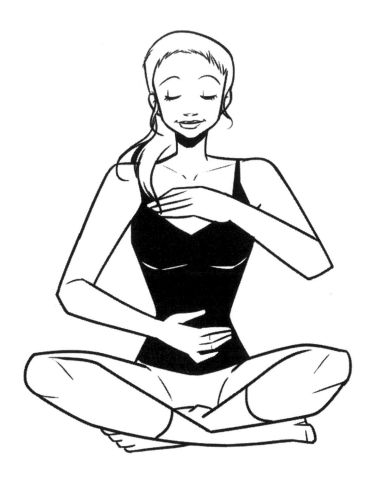

"Strive for deeper,
slower and quieter breaths."

- Dr. Andrew Weil, Director of the Arizona Center for
Integrative Medicine at the University of Arizona

93
Secret

JUST BREATHE.

At a nutrition school live event, I had the chance of a lifetime to hear Dr. Andrew Weil speak. Not only is he a brilliant naturopathic doctor and teacher, but he is also filled with humor and helpful advice. He stressed the effectiveness of mindful, controlled breathing techniques as a useful tool to reduce stress.

He taught us this simple breathing technique that can be used throughout the day. This is the 4-7-8 exercise:

- Exhale completely through your mouth, making a whoosh sound.
- Close your mouth and inhale quietly through your nose to a mental count of **four.**
- Hold your breath for a count of **seven.**
- Exhale completely through your mouth, making a whoosh sound to a count of **eight**.
- This is one breath. Now inhale again and repeat the cycle three more times for a total of four breaths.

Note that you always inhale quietly through your nose and exhale audibly through your mouth. Exhalation takes twice as long as inhalation. The actual time you spend on each step is not important; the ratio of 4:7:8 is important. With practice, you can slow it all down and get used to inhaling and exhaling more and more deeply.

This exercise is a natural tranquilizer for the nervous system. Do it at least twice a day. If you feel a little lightheaded when you first breathe this way, don't be concerned; it will pass.

Once you develop this technique by practicing it every day, it will be a very useful tool that you will always have with you. **Whenever anything upsetting happens, stop and breathe before you react.** Use it whenever you feel stressed. Use it to help you fall asleep. **This exercise cannot be recommended too highly.** Everyone can benefit from it.

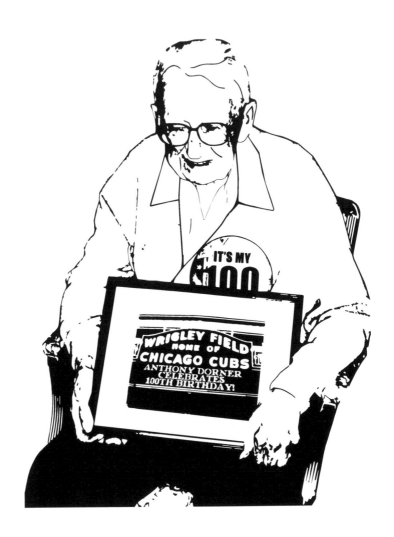

What is your goal?

My grandfather's goal was to live to
100 and he exceeded it!

94

Secret

"LOVE MEANS ALWAYS SAYING YOU'RE SORRY AND NEVER GOING TO BED MAD." - TONY DORNER

My grandfather lived until the age of 101 and his marriage lasted almost 72 years until his wife passed away. The key to his long marriage? Never going to bed mad. The key to his life? Letting go of things that could have kept him up at night.

He also knew how to relax. He used to say: "When its 4 its time to pour", and would proceed to make a perfect Manhattan. He knew when it was time to leave behind the problems of the day and switch gears so he could enjoy the evening.

I had the chance to hear Dan Buettner, author of *The Blue Zones*, speak at an IIN live event about how he traveled the world learning the key characteristics of those living in communities that have the highest proportions of people living past the age of 100. Many of these I saw reflected in my grandfather, and I'm sharing them now with you:

1. **Keep moving**—love being active and strive for an active lifestyle. Love what gets you moving.
2. **Eat less**—eat until you are about 80% full. Use small plates.
3. **Limit meat and processed foods**—load up on local, seasonal fruits, and veggies from your town.
4. **Have a drink**—one beer, wine, or spirit. Happy hour has benefits.
5. **Live with purpose**—happiness comes from having a clear goal.
6. **Relieve stress**—reduce noise and embrace quiet time without electronics.
7. **Believe in a higher power** or spiritual practice.
8. **Loving and supporting your family takes priority** above all else.
9. **Surround yourself with those who live by the principles above.**

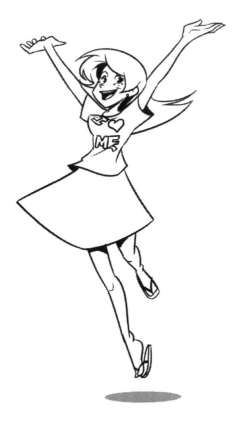

"You can't force a rosebud to blossom by hitting it with a hammer."

When loving someone through an illness,
remember this advice from Dr. Lissa Rankin.

95

Secret

BELIEVE ANYTHING
IS POSSIBLE.

Patients need hope and encouragement, not just medications, treatments and a list of statistics. If you or someone you love has just been diagnosed with a disease, even a rare disease, you should be aware that there is such a thing as spontaneous remission that is often brought on by self-induced healing.

Dr. Lissa Rankin, author of *Mind Over Medicine*, is emphatic about the idea that if patients learn the story of even one person who has beaten the odds, it offers the patient a level of hope they may not have had without it. She encourages patients to look for stories, "*The Spontaneous Remission Project* is a database maintained by the Institute of Noetic Sciences, with more than 3500 studies in the medical literature of patients betterment of seemingly "incurable" diseases."

Dr. Rankin passionately advocates this six-step process to mind-over-matter healing:

1. **Believe** in your body's potential to be well.
2. Get **support** from others who believe in your potential to be well. Dismiss anyone who doesn't.
3. **Intuition**—learn to listen to what your body is telling you.
4. **Diagnose**—get a diagnosis and be proactive about treatment.
5. **Prescribe**—what does your body need to heal?
6. **Surrender** your illness to a higher power, and then go back to step 1.

We don't need to mislead each other or be unrealistic about our health. But we do know belief and taking action DO go a long way in the self-induced healing process.

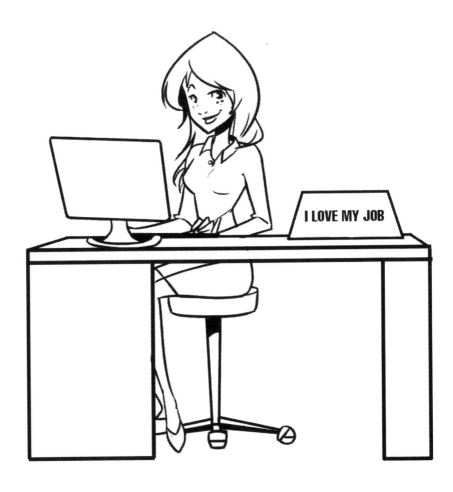

Build a healthy resume.

96

Secret

LOVE THE WORK YOU DO!

Let's get real. Do you love your job? Most of the time I just hear people complaining.

Let's explore. Is there a way to love the work you do? Or are there ways to love being in the space, around the people or at least the lunch breaks? How's the view?

Think about this, most people spend about forty hours a week at work. That is a lot of time to spend either loving or hating your job.

The most important thing is to have the desire and courage to know that you can improve your situation and end up in a happier and healthier environment. If you can't stand your current job—then start updating your resumé. Set some boundaries about your work-load.

There are ways to make your current work space better by clearing off your desk, and perhaps adding some music, plants or photos to make your work space more inviting. These types of changes will enhance your mood and your healthy mindset.

I can tell you from experience that it is never too late! I went back to school and opened my electrolysis practice at 30. Then I went back to school and opened my coaching practice at 40! At 42 I became an author! I am certain there is more to come!

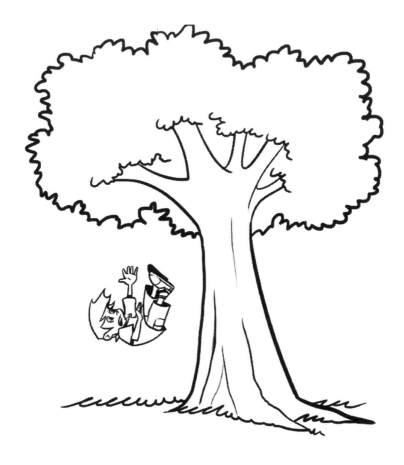

Don't spend the day thinking about things that may never happen.

This was key for me to becoming a less worried and more confident mother.

97

Secret

THINK POSITIVE THOUGHTS

Negative thoughts are toxic to our bodies. They can fill us with fear, anxiety, stress, and make you feel chaotic, which can be harmful to our health.

Pay attention to how you are thinking. When negative thoughts bother you, release them. Then think positive thoughts and write them down to create awareness. This will help you flip the switch from negative to positive.

Also practice this exercise taught by author and television personality Iyanla Vanzant, a speaker at IIN. **Every time a negative thought enters her mind, she thinks, "cancel, cancel" until it passes.** Or create your own mantra of strength and kindness.

Committing to the "cancel, cancel" habit will free your heart and mind to move forward in life. **Time to think positive.**

Some of my favorite reversal thoughts are:

Start over, start over.

It's okay now, it's okay.

Let it go, let it go.

Faith over fear, focus over fear.

My body is healthy, happy, and whole.

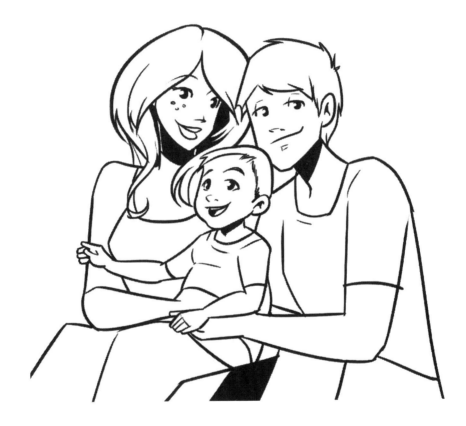

98

Secret

I LOVE YOU AND
I HOPE YOU DANCE.

All you need is hope to get started on your healing journey.

And we all know that love can be the best medicine. Many researchers and practicing medical doctors have explored the importance of love and hope in the healing process. What have they found? **It's never too late to love yourself and enjoy hope's healing powers.**

In a lecture by Dr. Bernie Siegel, noted surgical oncologist, he shared a simple and yet powerful example about four new cancer drugs that came out. They began with the letters E, P, O and H, and were called the EPOH protocol. He explained that one of the doctors looked at the letters and thought: "Why don't I turn the letters around and make them spell HOPE?" After he did this, they noticed that more patients in his program responded to this treatment than to the doctors who were giving it labeled as EPOH. What was the difference? The patients were given HOPE.

Dr. Siegel went on to say, "If I were empowered to do one thing, **it would be to see that every child felt loved.** When that happens, wars cease, addictions and self destructive behavior end, and the world becomes a meaningful place to live. Love can change the world."

No matter where you are in your healing process I offer you hope and I love you.

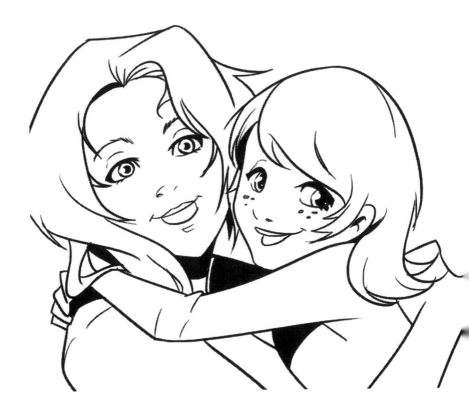

I forgive you, Mom.

99

Secret

FORGIVENESS IS THE BLESSING YOU GIVE YOURSELF.

I was sitting in the large auditorium at a recent IIN conference. Out walked a beautiful, sassy, intelligent woman named Dr. Christiane Northrup. I had no idea at the time that this woman would have such an immense impact on my life and I hope that this will support you too.

She made her point clear. Forgive your mother. She did the best she could. At first, I just felt numb. She went on to explain that how we **feel about our mothers is at the root of our hearts and ability to live and heal in our daily lives.**

She repeated: Your mother did the best she could with the tools she had. That's when the hot tears started streaming down my face. I am not sure I could breathe at this point, I sat there frozen.

At that moment, all I could think of was—**my mother did the best that she could** and finally I realized it was enough.

Somewhere during Christiane's talk, I finally embraced that I was going to forgive myself. **I am a mother and I am doing the best I can with the tools that I have.** I find it so important to be adding more tools every day.

Oprah Winfrey offered an easier definition for the word forgiveness that I would like to share with you, "**Forgiveness is giving up the hope that the past could have been any different.**"

Forgiveness is freedom.

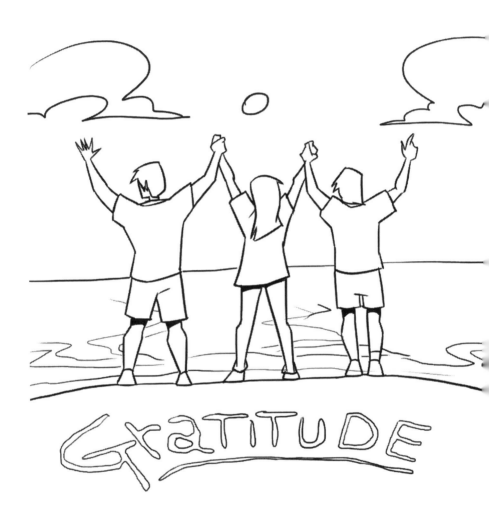

100

Secret

EVERY DAY IS THE BEST DAY OF YOUR LIFE.

Gratitude, the heart-based art of being thankful and appreciative, draws joy and comfort into your life.

Being grateful for all things, big or small, is good for more than your attitude, it's good for your health, too. Here's how it can help:

- Gratitude reduces stress
- Gratitude improves relationships
- Gratitude increases resilience
- Gratitude makes us happier

Besides reducing stress, research shows that practicing gratitude daily, maybe through writing in a gratitude journal, helps people achieve **higher levels of alertness, enthusiasm, determination, attentiveness, and energy.** Feelings of gratitude actually alter your body chemistry and produce feel-good hormones like serotonin.

According to Robert Emmons, renowned research expert on the benefits of gratitude, people who practice gratitude regularly report becoming 20-25% happier with their lives. They can also reduce their level of the stress hormone cortisol by 23%, boost their immune system, and balance their mood swings.

What are you grateful for?

I encourage you to make a list of three things you are grateful for everyday. The longer you practice this, the more your health and happiness levels will increase. This has been an especially helpful exercise for my clients with anxiety and depression disorders.

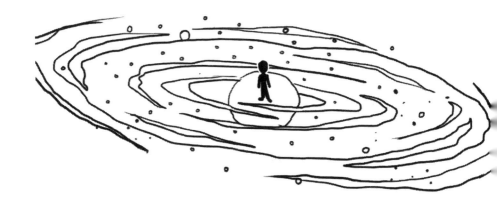

Look in the mirror—do you see it?

The most beautiful person in the world

I love this lesson, a lasting memory of
my grandmother, Anne Soens.

101

Secret

YOU ARE THE SECRET.

Your consciousness is filled with endless possibilities to change your life.

Deepak Chopra, one of my teachers at nutrition school, explained that your body and mind are expressions of consciousness and only consciousness can change the mind and body. It is a field of infinite possibilities.

Meaning? **Our minds and bodies are connected deeply.** Through this connection, and by understanding and honoring it, we hold the power to shift our thoughts and physically shift our lives.

What miracles do you yearn for? You hold the power of change within you.

Life is a gift. What you do with it is your choice. You have what it takes to live your happiest and healthiest life.

You are the gift.
You are the secret.
You are the star in your play.
You are the music worth dancing to.
You are the sun that shines.
You are the moonlight to rest under.

You are the goals you set.
You are the steps that you take.
You are the decisions that you make.

You have the power to stand up for yourself.

You are enough.

You can do the job.

You only live once.
You are the secret.

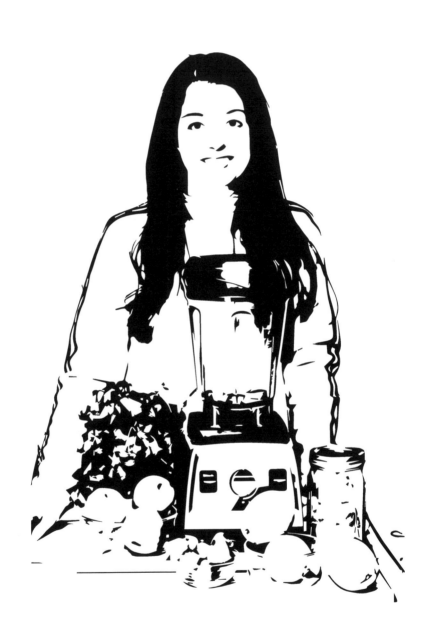

MY JOURNEY LIVING THE SECRETS

I believe that I have always been on a passionate, adventurous and spiritual journey. I have a huge heart, love of education, enthusiasm, compassion for all people, and a "do your best" mentality.

During my experience at Integrative Nutrition®, I was astounded at the level of speakers that we were exposed to such as Deepak Chopra, Arianna Huffington and Dr. Mark Hyman. Many times I would be listening to a lecture and have to stop and pinch myself because I was so honored to be learning from the top doctors and educators in the field. I am proud to say that **I fully invested and intensively completed the program** by listening to every lecture, devouring every book and article, completing every assignment no matter how large or small, and most importantly absorbed much wisdom. This allowed me to start making immediate changes in every aspect of my life.

I researched more than 100 dietary theories, from A to Z, from the Atkins diet to the Zone diet. At the end, I was encouraged to find what would work for me specifically. I've always loved food and preparing it for others, but now I have a profound respect for it and its potential to transform our health.

It was a tremendous joy to go through school and be able to share my experiences with my electrolysis clients. I now had a solid foundation in which to really guide them. Many of my clients suffer from PCOS (polycystic ovarian syndrome) and it was fulfilling to be able to help them manage some of their symptoms. Some clients found that by changing their eating habits they were even finally able to get pregnant. Since women with PCOS struggle with the effects of insulin resistance, a carefully managed diet could help control the symptoms. It was amazing to watch the transformations that my clients were experiencing which helped them much more than I could with my electrolysis equipment alone.

I find it exciting that in my forties I have found a whole new set of friends and colleagues that have the same priorities and interests. We are a community of people from all over the world who came together to support each other during a time when we were all in transition and experimenting with ways to change our lives. These relationships have continued and deepened. We laugh, we cry, and we understand one another in such a unique way.

Perhaps the most unbelievable changes were to my health.
When I began school, I didn't realize how unhealthy I actually was, until I started to feel so much better. I suffered from chronic fatigue, migraines, irritable bowel syndrome, brain fog, allergies, and chronic neck and shoulder pain.

I worked on cleaning out the toxins in my body and my life.
I learned to love to eat clean. Through this cleansing process, I began noticing unimaginable improvements in my health. I had more energy, my migraines lessened, my irritable bowel syndrome was erased, and the pain that had been aggravating me for so long was going away! I hadn't lived a day in over 10 years without significant pain in my neck, shoulders, and back, and now it was gone—what a miracle.

I also became more aware of professional and personal relationships that weren't moving in the right direction, and released them. This is not to say it was easy or always very pretty. I had a tendency to care too much about what others thought of me, which caused me to stay in unhealthy relationships. It was like I had been lugging around a purse with an accumulation of many years' worth of loose change, receipts, and random junk, and I decided it was high time to clean it all out.

Evaluating my priorities became a priority. I started re-allocating the amount of time that I devoted to each of the essential areas of my life. I used to work seven days a week, essentially putting my relationships last. I spread myself too thin, volunteering to help everyone else—even people I would hire to help me. I was so afraid to cut my hours and put time with my family first. When I did, a strange thing happened—clients scheduled their appointments around MY available hours. Now I don't work most nights, I don't work Sundays, and I took my first real vacation in 12 years. It is a start!

With the major changes I was making in my career, I also wanted to strengthen my financial future and make it a primary focus.
I definitely inherited the love of finance and a small obsession with following the stock market from my grandfather. With some solid advice from our instructor, Manisha Thakor, I worked out new systems and plans to save for a home, retirement, and my son's education. It's amazing what can be done with a little information and a lot of determination. Now for the first time, I feel secure knowing I have a plan in which I know I am investing in myself for the long term.

I used to have a list of excuses why I didn't have time to exercise, and now I know it's something worth making time for. I love exploring yoga, swimming, running in Central Park, riding bikes, roller-blading, doing some T-25, Zumba, and playing with my son in an active way I hadn't in the past. It feels fantastic!

Spirituality has always been a focus in my life but for many years I hadn't found a spiritual home/family. I spent the year visiting many different churches all over the city to find one that was the best fit for our family. Our new spiritual home has brought many blessings into our lives, and we stay dedicated to going to church every Sunday and being active members of the community. It feels great to have this support and love in our lives.

Through my work, I also have the distinct pleasure of meeting and sharing with people of all faiths right in my own office! **I call it my mini UN.** Honestly, I feel like we could solve world peace in my office—as all religions have something special and lovely to offer its followers. I am so blessed to practice in New York City with such a unique and diverse set of clients.

With my newfound sense of who I am, **I was inspired to renovate my home.** I had recently embraced feng shui after attending a lecture at IIN. Since home and office spaces are major elements of focus in the practice of feng shui, it led to me painting my living space with "Lynne colors." I hired a client, Dawn of *Paradigm Interior Design*, to pick the colors from some of my favorite beach photos that another client (the amazing photographer Sari Goodfriend) had given me. The beautiful beachy colors really inspire me. I also filled my kitchen with fresh organic foods and brought music into this space as well. I stocked up on amazing smelling organic soaps and cleansers, and bought the best cotton sheets and towels for ultimate comfort and coziness. As I cleaned out each box, bag, drawer, and my extensive medicine cabinet, I felt refreshed and renewed. My new home is now organized with my life's essentials: music, healthy foods, creative art supplies, fuzzy towels, sturdy shoes, plants, and fresh flowers next to my bed-and love.

Taking the time to revamp my style was perhaps the most fun! I decided that since looking good is a part of feeling good, it was time to make some changes. It was time to get rid of the low-rise jeans, way-too high heels, and ill-fitting sweaters. I hired a stylist, Natalie Tincher of Buttoned Up Style, to help me. She came in and did a Closet Consultation, where we went through recycled all the clothes that didn't look good or fit right (even the expensive ones with tags on them). Natalie took me shopping to help me find what looked good based on my needs, style, body type, and coloring. This was such an incredible process and I finally feel good in my jeans!

The most meaningful changes were what I experienced as a mom. I implemented some difficult advice I heard from my trusted friend, Peggy: **let go.** I don't have to do it all perfectly. Being the best mom I could be IS enough. I committed to really listening to my son's needs. Now I am dedicated to clearing my schedule for him to enjoy running full-speed in the park, coaching little league, singing songs at the top of our lungs, full-out dancing no matter where we are, coloring our best masterpieces, or laughing at *Captain Underpants* books. **Now I really feel like I'm living in the sweet spot of motherhood.**

Most recently, I decided that I was finally willing to let go of my past and my insecurities and make space for the **opportunity to meet a partner.** Only time will tell the rewards and benefits from this leap, and I believe the future is bright. I am ready to give my heart to this new adventure.

As a result of my journey at IIN and all of the surprising, beautiful changes it has inspired, I found exactly what I was looking for: I love the simplicity of my home. I love that my relationships are stronger and authentic. I love my job: my clients, my hours, and helping people start their own journey toward changing and loving their lives. I love how I look and feel. **And now, I am an Author!** My journey at IIN gave me the courage to dream big and provided the structure I needed to make those dreams happen. If I can hope for **one more** positive action to come from my experience at IIN, it's that **by writing this book, my work might be the drop that begins the ripple of change in my readers.**

P.S. In case you're curious, after all my experimentation with dietary theories, I decided it wasn't in my Bio-individuality to be a super-strict vegan angel. I still eat meat, drink coffee, and love my organic dark chocolate stash. On special occasions, I enjoy a few cocktails with friends, especially when rocking some karaoke! **The key for me is enjoying as much of life as possible while striving to find a healthy balance.**

Personally, I feel better in my skin than ever before. **I am a part of something so immense, yet so deeply personal; and I will always be thankful that I learned these secrets that I can share with you.**

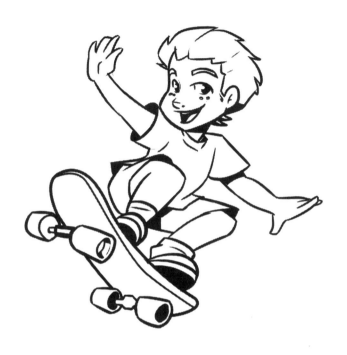

Put your heart into it and enjoy the ride!

ABOUT THE AUTHOR

Lynne Dorner is a graduate of the Institute for Integrative Nutrition (IIN) and is a Health and Wellness Specialist who creates an environment in which her clients transform and thrive in their daily lives. She specializes in working with health professionals and educates them on ways to incorporate holistic, natural healing methods into their everyday lives and their medical practices.

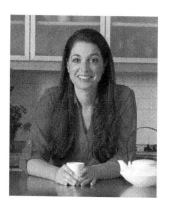

Her ultimate passion lies in serving others. She finds no greater joy than helping her clients overcome obstacles and excuses to achieve success after success. Lynne is passionate about goal setting and clean eating to bring about long-lasting and drastic results.

Her path to this career began with 10+ years of experience as a top electrologist, where she supports her clients in permanent hair removal, often caused by underlying health and hormonal issues. Throughout the process she works with her clients to overcome any self-esteem issues related to their embarrassing and unwanted hair.

Lynne has her thriving Electrolysis and Health Coaching practices in Manhattan, where she also resides with her son.

RECLAIM YOUR HEALTH

Clean eating starts with a clean plate.
Learn how to build one!

Lynne Dorner is the founder and program director at CleanEatingPrograms.com. She loves teaching her clients to prepare and eat organic, local, seasonal, simple and nutritious recipes without missing out on all their favorite flavors while reducing junk food cravings.

She created a team of experts to support both beginner and advanced clean eaters.

If you suffer from allergies, digestive issues, candida overgrowth, skin conditions, diabetes, or autoimmune conditions, I encourage you to seek out a safe, supervised, gentle clean eating program that focuses on whole foods and reducing allergens.

For more information on the benefits of clean eating visit:

www.CleanEatingPrograms.com

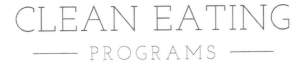

JOIN THE JOURNEY

For more information on enrolling
at Integrative Nutrition® head over to:

www.LynneDorner.com
-or-
www.IntegrativeNutrition.com

(877) 733-1520

Lynne Dorner is a proud Ambassador of IIN® and she would
love to explore the possibilities with you.

You may contact her at **lynnedorner@gmail.com** and put in
the subject field "I want to change my life!"

101+ Secrets from Nutrition School will be available for bulk
discounts for schools, churches, hospitals and book clubs.

Lynne is also available for live speaking engagements,
cooking demos, webinars, and teleclasses.

www.NutritionSchoolSecrets.com

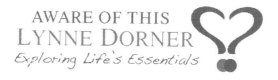

Marilena Minucci, MS, CHC, BCC

As creator of the **Quantum Coaching Method**™, and author of **Quantum Coaching Questions**, Marilena Minucci offers health coaches and other wellness professionals a dynamic way to work more deeply and effectively with their clients while at the same time enhancing their own individual wellbeing. She shares her mastery in challenging clients to examine old patterns and beliefs that keep them stuck, to end cycles of self-sabotage, to identify meaningful goals, and to design effective strategies to move ahead and create the more fulfilling lives they desire.

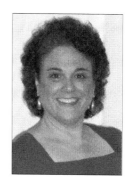

In addition to her advanced studies in Counseling and Psychology and board certification as a wellness coach, Marilena is a graduate of the **Institute for Integrative Nutrition**® (IIN) in New York where she has continued to serve as a mentor and instructor for over 10 years. She is a 2013 recipient of the IIN Health Leadership Award.

www.QuantumCoachingMethod.com

To our nana, Pauline,
who passed away during
the creation of this book.

You filled our lives
with light and are
missed greatly!

Love,
Ali & Drew Johnson

PS. Lynne wants you to meet up
with her grandparents in heaven!

REFERENCES

Some of the information contained in this book was adapted from the curriculum of the Institute for Integrative Nutrition® ©2012 Integrative Nutrition Inc.

The terms, Institute for Integrative Nutrition®, Integrative Nutrition®, IIN®, Bio-individuality™, and Primary Food™ are trademarks that are owned and/or in use by Integrative Nutrition Inc.

Secret 1:   Rosenthal, Joshua. *Integrative Nutrition: Feed Your Hunger for Health and Happiness.* New York, NY: Integrative Nutrition Pub., 2014. 35-39.

Secret 2:   Rosenthal, J. *Integrative Nutrition.* 142-164.

Secret 7:   *Overweight in the Military.* Rep. Health Care Survey of DoD Beneficiaries, Jan. 2005. Web. 9 Nov. 2014. <http://www.tricare.mil/survey/hcsurvey/default.cfm>.

Secret 11: Munro, Dan. "Annual U.S. Healthcare Spending Hits $3.8 Trillion." Web post. *Forbes.* 2 Feb. 2014. 10 Nov. 2014. <http://www.forbes.com/sites/danmunro/2014/02/02/annual-u-s-healthcare-spending-hits-3-8-trillion/>.

"Historical Data." *National Health Expenditure Data.* Centers for Medicare & Medicaid Services, 7 Jan. 2014. 10 Nov. 2014. <http://www.cms.gov/Research-Statistics-Data-and-Systems/Statistics-Trends-and-Reports/NationalHealthExpendData/NationalHealthAccountsHistorical.html>.

World Health Organization. "Life Expectancy and Mortality." *World Health Statistics 2013.* Geneva: World Health Organization, 2013. 49-60. Available at: http://www.who.int/gho/publications/world_health_statistics/EN_WHS2013_Full.pdf

Secret 12: Tatchell, Peter. "The Oxygen Crisis." http://www.theguardian.com/commentisfree/2008/aug/13/carbonemissions.climatechange. The Guardian, 13 Aug. 2008. 10 Nov. 2014.

Secret 18: Hyman, Mark. "How Diet Soda Makes You Fat (and Other Food and Diet Industry Secrets)." Web post. *Dr. Mark Hyman.* 22 Feb. 2013. 10 Nov. 2014. <http://drhyman.com/blog/2013/02/15/how-diet-soda-makes-you-fat-and-other-food-and-diet-industry-secrets/>.

Hyman, Mark. *The Blood Sugar Solution: The Ultrahealthy Program for Losing Weight, Preventing Disease, and Feeling Great Now!* New York, NY: Little, Brown, 2012.

Associated Press. "WHO: 5 Percent of Calories Should Be from Sugar." *USA Today.* N.p., 5 Mar. 2014. Web. 10 Nov. 2014. <http://www.usatoday.com/story/news/world/2014/03/05/five-percent-of-calories-should-be-from-sugar/6097623/>.

Secret 18: U.S. Department of Agriculture. "Profiling Food Consumption in America." *Agriculture Fact Book.* Washington, DC: Office of Communications, U.S. Dept. of Agriculture, 2002. 20-22. Available at: http://www.usda.gov

Secret 19: U.S. Department of Agriculture and U.S. Department of Health and Human Services. Dietary Guidelines for Americans, 2010. 7th Edition, Washington, DC: U.S. Government Printing Office, December 2010. Available at: www.dietaryguidelines.gov

Secret 28: No Free Lunch, 2012. Web. <nofreelunch.org>.

Secret 31: Mercola, Joseph. "Can Juicing Really Lead to Happiness?" Web post. *Mercola.com.* N.p., 16 Apr. 2009. Web. 10 Nov. 2014. <http://articles.mercola.com/sites/articles/archive/2009/04/16/can-juicing-really-lead-to-happiness.aspx>.

Secret 34: Randolph, Theron G., and Ralph W. Moss. *An Alternative Approach to Allergies: The New Field of Clinical Ecology Unravels the Environmental Causes of Mental and Physical Ills.* New York: Lippincott & Crowell, 1980.

Secret 38: Fallon, Sally, and Mary G. Enig. "The Skinny on Fats." Weblog post. *The Weston A. Price Foundation.* N.p., 1 Jan. 2000. Web. 10 Nov. 2014. <http://www.westonaprice.org/health-topics/the-skinny-on-fats/>.

Secret 40: Rosenthal, J. *Integrative Nutrition.* 111-113.

Secret 42: Environmental Working Group. 2014 *Shopper's Guide to Pesticides in Produce.* Washington, D.C. : Environmental Working Group, 2014. <http://www.ewg.org/foodnews/>.

Secret 46: Lyman, Howard F., and Glen Merzer. *Mad Cowboy.: Plain Truth from the Cattle Rancher Who Won't Eat Meat.* New York: Scribner, 1998.

Secret 48: Keniger LE, Gaston KJ, Irvine KN, Fuller RA. What are the Benefits of Interacting with Nature? International Journal of Environmental Research and Public Health. 2013; 10(3):913-935. Available at http://www.ncbi.nlm.nih.gov/pmc/articles/PMC3709294/

Many studies are also summarized at: College of the Environment. "Mental Health & Function." Weblog post. *Green Cities: Good Health.* University of Washington, 11 Sept. 2014. Web. 10 Nov. 2014. <http://depts.washington.edu/hhwb/Thm_Mental.html>.

Secret 49: *See secret 48*

Secret 50: Robert Notter, IIN CONFERENCE appearance

Secret 51: National Center for Chronic Disease Prevention and Health Promotion. *Trans Fats: The Facts.* Atlanta: Centers for Disease Control and Prevention, 2014. Available at http://www.cdc.gov/nutrition/everyone/basics/fat/transfat.html

U.S. Food and Drug Administration. "FDA Targets Trans Fat in Processed Foods." Weblog post. *Consumer Updates*. N.p., 7 Nov. 2013. Web. <http://www.fda.gov/ForConsumers/ConsumerUpdates/ucm372915.htm>.

Leary, Warren E. "Genetic Engineering of Crops Can Spread Allergies, Study Shows." *The New York Times*. N.p., 14 Mar. 1996. Web. 10 Nov. 2014. <http://www.nytimes.com/1996/03/14/us/genetic-engineering-of-crops-can-spread-allergies-study-shows.html>.

Union of Concerned Scientists. "Genetic Engineering Risks and Impacts." Weblog post. N.p., n.d. Web. 10 Nov. 2014. <www.ucsusa.org/food_and_agriculture/our-failing-food-system/genetic-engineering/risks-of-genetic-engineering.html>.

"Farmed Salmon and Human Health." *Pure Salmon Campaign - Raising the Standards for Farm-Raised Fish*. N.p., n.d. Web. 10 Nov. 2014. <http://www.puresalmon.org/human_health.html>.

For references regarding soda and sugar see Secret 18.
For references regarding factory-farmed meat see Secret 46.

Secret 55: Grøntved A, Hu FB. Television Viewing and Risk of Type 2 Diabetes, Cardiovascular Disease, and All-Cause Mortality: A Meta-analysis. JAMA. 2011;305(23):2448-2455. doi:10.1001/jama.2011.812. Available at http://jama.jamanetwork.com/article.aspx?articleid=900893

See also Hyman, M. *The Blood Sugar Solution*. 22.

Secret 60: Marketdata. *The U.S. Weight Loss & Diet Control Market*. Rep. N.p., 1 Mar. 2013.

See also data summarized at http://www.worldometers.info/weight-loss/.

Secret 62: Robbins, John. *Diet for a New America: How Your Food Choices Affect Your Health, Your Happiness, and the Future of Life on Earth*. Tiburon: H J Kramer, 2012. 173.

Robbins, John. "The Truth About Calcium and Osteoporosis." Weblog post. *Food Matters*. Permacology Productions, 24 Nov. 2009. Web. 10 Nov. 2014. <http://foodmatters.tv/articles-1/the-truth-about-calcium-and-osteoporosis>.

Secret 68: Batmanghelidj, F. *Water: For Health, for Healing, for Life: You're Not Sick, You're Thirsty!* New York: Warner, 2003.

See also http://www.watercure.com

Secret 69: See Dr. John Douillard's website www.lifespa.com.

Secret 70: Colbin, Annemarie. Headaches An Article by Annemarie Colbin. And What to do about them. <http://www.foodandhealing.com/>

Secret 72: "Heart Disease and Oral Health." Weblog post. *National Institute of Dental and Craniofacial Research*. N.p., 30 July 2014. Web. 10 Nov. 2014. <http://www.nidcr.nih.gov/oralhealth/Topics/HeartDisease/>.

Secret 74: *See Secret 62*.

Secret 76: Siegel, Bernie S., and Cynthia Hurn. *The Art of Healing: Uncovering Your Inner Wisdom and Potential for Self-healing*. California: New World Library, 2013.

Secret 78: Smith, Lindsey. "Food Mood Girl." Web. 10 Nov. 2014. <http://foodmoodgirl.com/>.

Secret 79: Gates, Donna. "Body Ecology Healthy Diet." *The Body Ecology Diet, The Healthy Diet and Nutritional Supplements Source*. Body Ecology Inc. Web. 10 Nov. 2014. <http://bodyecology.com/>.

Secret 81: Douillard, John. "Oil for Your Ears and Nose (Nasya)." Weblog post. *Dr. Douillard's LifeSpa*. 17 Dec. 2008. Web. 10 Nov. 2014. <http://lifespa.com/oil-for-your-ears-and-nose/>.

Hyman, Mark. "Supporting Your Immune System When You May Need It Most." Weblog post. *Dr. Mark Hyman*. 19 Oct. 2014. 10 Nov. 2014. <http://drhyman.com/blog/2010/11/18/supporting-your-immune-system/>.

Secret 82: Katz, David, M.D. "Attention Deficit Disorder: Ritalin Or Recess?" *The Huffington Post*. TheHuffingtonPost.com, 07 May 2010. Web. 10 Nov. 2014. <http://www.huffingtonpost.com/david-katz-md/attention-deficit-disorde_b_541581.html>.

Jarrett, Olga S., Darlene M. Maxwell, Carrie Dickerson, Pamela Hoge, Gwen Davies, and Amy Yetley. "Impact of Recess on Classroom Behavior: Group Effects and Individual Differences." *The Journal of Educational Research* 92.2 (1998): 121-26.

Secret 84: Bratman, Steven. *Health Food Junkies: Overcoming the Obsession with Healthful Eating*. New York: Broadway, 2000.

Secret 95: Rankin, Lissa. Lecture at IIN conference.

"Is There Scientific Proof That We Can Heal Ourselves?" *Visual Meditation*. N.p., 21 Sept. 2014. Web. 10 Nov. 2014. <http://visualmeditation.co/is-there-scientific-proof-we-can-heal-ourselves-lissa-rankin-md/>.

Secret 100: Emmons, Robert A. Thanks!: *How the New Science of Gratitude Can Make You Happier*. Boston: Houghton Mifflin, 2007.

General Sources/Further Reading

www.nutritionschoolsecrets.com/references

www.health.gov

RECOMMENDED READING

Louise L. Hay, *You Can Heal Your Life*

Dr. William Davis, *Wheat Belly*

Thich Nhat Hanh, *Peace Is Every Step*

Dr. Bernie S. Siegel, *A Book of Miracles*

Haville Hendrix, Ph.D. *Getting the Love You Want*

Gary Chapman, *The Five Love Languages*

Ban Buettner, *The Blue Zones*

Johnna Albi and Catherine Walthers, *Greens Glorious Greens*

Joshua Rosenthal, *Integrative Nutrition*

Dr. Christiane Northrup, *Women's Bodies, Women's Wisdom*

Dr. Andrew Weil, *Healthy Aging*

Arianna Huffington, *Thrive*

Nina Planck, *Real Food*

Alice Waters, *The Art of Simple Food*

Jennifer Esposito, *Jennifer's Way*

Venus Williams, *Come to Win*

Iyanla Vanzant, *Forgiveness*

Additional reading or information:

Rhonda Britten, *Fearless Living*

Eckhart Tolle, *A New Earth, Awakening Your Life's Purpose*

Dr John Sarno, *Heal Your Back*

Elizabeth Gilbert, *Eat Pray Love*

Daniel Vitalis, *Rewild Yourself!*

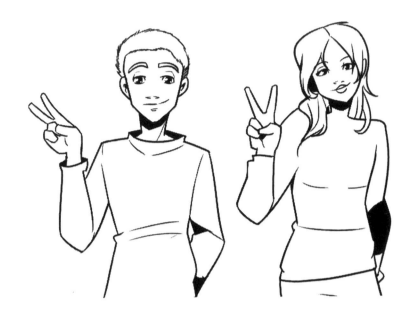

"*I really do want world peace.*"

- Gracie Hart, *Miss Congeniality*

Made in the USA
Middletown, DE
01 July 2016